£11.95
D

POCKET CONSULTANT

Haematology

B.T. Colvin
MA MRCP FRCPath
Senior Lecturer in Haematology

A.C. Newland
MA MRCP MRCPath
Senior Lecturer in Haematology

Both of The London Hospital and Medical College
Whitechapel
London

Blackwell Scientific Publications

OXFORD LONDON EDINBURGH

BOSTON PALO ALTO MELBOURNE

Editorial offices:
Osney Mead, Oxford OX2 0EL
(*Orders*: Tel. 0865 240201)
8 John Street, London WC1N 2ES
23 Ainslie Place, Edinburgh
EH3 6AJ
3 Cambridge Center, Suite 208
Cambridge, Massachusetts
02142, USA
667 Lytton Avenue, Palo Alto
California 94301, USA
107 Barry Street, Carlton
Victoria 3053, Australia

First published 1988

Set by Times Graphic,
Singapore, and printed and bound
in Great Britain by
Billings & Sons Ltd,
Worcester

DISTRIBUTORS
USA
Year Book Medical
Publishers
200 North LaSalle Street
Chicago, Illinois 60601
(*Orders*: Tel. 312 726-
9733)

Canada
The C.V. Mosby Company
5240 Finch Avenue East,
Scarborough, Ontario
(*Orders*: Tel. 416-298-
1588)

Australia
Blackwell Scientific
Publications
(Australia) Pty Ltd
107 Barry Street
Carlton, Victoria 3053
(*Orders*: Tel. (03) 347 0300)

British Library
Cataloguing in Publication
Data

Colvin, B.T.
Haematology. — (Pocket
Consultant)
1. Haematology
I. Title II. Newland, A.C.
616.1'5 RB145

ISBN 0-632-01092-4

Contents

Preface

This book is a practical account of the investigation and management of haematological disorders for the non-specialist, designed to assist the everyday practice of haematology in a district general hospital. It is not intended to replace the large standard textbooks which usually contain a wealth of theoretical and scientific detail which may be of limited value at the bedside.

The text is divided into two clinical introductory sections followed by a summary of laboratory haematology and a more detailed account of haematological practice. We hope that this will assist the reader to find the answer to a problem, whether related to laboratory investigation or clinical work, without having to read more that a page or two of print.

It is also hoped that medical students wishing to gain further insight into the subject and trainees revising for postgraduate examinations may find this synopsis of value.

1 Clinical introduction

1 Clinical introduction

1.1 Anaemia

Anaemia is usually defined as a reduction in haemoglobin concentration below values adjusted for age and sex, which are given on p. 39. The clinical consequences of anaemia depend on:

- Haemoglobin concentration.
- The rapidity with which the anaemia has developed.
- The age of the patient.
- The compensatory mechanisms of the body.

For instance, the anaemic patient with haematinic deficiency may be remarkably well despite a very low haemoglobin concentration while acute intravascular haemolysis may have serious consequences. Paradoxically, the patient who has just suffered a catastrophic gastrointestinal haemorrhage may have a normal or near normal haemoglobin concentration in the blood still circulating.

The clinical effects of anaemia are:

- Pallor.
- Weakness.
- Tiredness.
- Shortness of breath, especially on exertion.
- Angina pectoris or intermittent claudication, usually in patients with occlusive vascular disease.
- General malaise.

Pallor of the mucous membranes is usually the only sign specifically due to the anaemia itself, but sometimes the spleen is just palpable in chronically anaemic patients. Anaemia should not be accepted as the cause of a palpable spleen without a thorough search for some other pathology.

1.2 Polycythaemia

Polycythaemia conventionally refers only to an excess of circulating red blood cells. The red blood cell count in health is affected by:

- Age.
- Sex.
- Altitude.

Typical effects of polycythaemia include:

- Headache or a feeling of fullness in the head.
- Tinnitus.
- Visual disturbance.
- Angina pectoris or intermittent claudication, usually in patients with occlusive vascular disease.
- Gout.
- Plethora.
- Central cyanosis in hypoxic patients.
- Generalized pruritus and splenic enlargement only occur in patients with polycythaemia rubra vera (p. 213).

In addition, patients with uncontrolled polycythaemia have an increased incidence of cardiovascular, cerebrovascular and peripheral vascular occlusion. Some polycythaemic patients are also hypertensive, and there is an increased incidence of peptic ulceration. Clinical examination may help to distinguish the different causes of polycythaemia not due to hypoxia.

Rarer cases of polycythaemia due to increased erythropoietin production may be revealed on examination:

- Kidneys — tumour or obstruction.
- Liver — tumour.
- Pelvis — uterine fibroids.
- Nervous system — cerebellar haemangioma.

Extremely rare causes, such as high-affinity haemoglobin, are usually diagnosed by exclusion followed by definitive laboratory tests, though age at presentation, a positive family history and lifelong symptoms give useful clues.

There is also a group of patients who on routine testing have apparent polycythaemia, but on further investigation prove to have a normal red cell mass together with a reduced plasma volume. This combination has been called 'stress' polycythaemia and tends to occur in overweight, tense individuals who smoke and are hypertensive.

1.3 Leucopenia

A reduction in white cell numbers is usually seen as an acquired phenomenon in adult life. The effects of severe granulocytopenia include:

- Localized bacterial infection.
- Septicaemia.
- Tissue necrosis, particularly within the mouth and around the anus.

Opportunistic infection is a major problem in haematology, especially in immunosuppressed patients, in whom lymphocyte numbers and function are also severely affected. Common sites of opportunistic infection include:

- Mouth and anus.
- Skin.
- Lungs.
- Urinary tract.
- Brain and meninges.
- Heart.

Infecting organisms often belong to one or more of the following groups:

- Bacteria (including tuberculosis).
- Fungi (especially Candida and Aspergillus).
- Herpes viruses including cytomegalovirus.
- *Pneumocystis carinii.*
- Mycoplasmas.

Infection and immunosuppression may also affect the development and course of graft versus host disease and the occurrence of secondary neoplasms.

1.4 Leucocytosis

An increase in the numbers of circulating white cells is usually a physiological reaction to some external stimulus. Leucocytosis can be associated with quite specific symptoms, e.g. the dramatic lymphocytosis sometimes seen in whooping cough and the mononucleosis characteristic of glandular fever.

The white cell mass must be very significantly elevated to produce clinical effects attributable to the leucocytes themselves.

- Lymph node and splenic enlargement commonly occur together in lymphoid neoplasms.
- In chronic myeloid proliferative states only the spleen is usually palpable.
- Gum hypertrophy and skin infiltration occasionally occur in monocytic leukaemias.
- Tumour may cause mediastinal obstruction or pressure damage to the nervous system in some lymphoid neoplasms.
- Bone and bone marrow necrosis can cause severe bone pain.

Where the white cell count is very high, usually above $200 \times 10^9/l$ in chronic granulocytic anaemia, interruption to blood flow may take place, resulting in

- Visual loss or other neurological signs.
- Dyspnoea.
- Priapism in the male.
- Gross splenic enlargement and infarction.

In acute leukaemia with or without a marked leucocytosis in the peripheral blood the clinical features are essentially those of functional leucopenia.

1.5 Thrombocytopenia

Although the normal platelet count is between 150 and $450 \times 10^9/l$, there is usually little clinical effect when counts are above $100 \times 10^9/l$. Between 50 and $100 \times 10^9/l$ abnormal bleeding may follow injury, but when the count falls below $50 \times 10^9/l$ there is a possibility of spontaneous bleeding, and at very low levels more serious problems such as cerebral haemorrhage may occur.

- Capillary oozing usually occurs from the nose, mouth, gums and skin.
- Menstruation may be difficult to control, but urinary and rectal bleeding, haematemesis and haemoptysis are less common.
- Fundal haemorrhage is often seen when the platelet count is very low.

The effect of severe thrombocytopenia on the skin is the most obvious clinical manifestation giving rise to:

- Purpura, petechial haemorrhages, ecchymoses and bruises.

Occasionally, symptoms or signs suggestive of thrombocytopenia may occur in the presence of a normal or near normal platelet count. Possible explanations then include:

- Telangiectasia — the capillary malformations may not be easy to see and there may not be a family history.
- Allergic purpura — Henoch–Schönlein.
- Meningococcal septicaemia.
- Scurvy.
- Von Willebrand's disease — there is a platelet functional defect whose nature can be confirmed by examining the various aspects of the factor VIII molecule.
- Rare congenital defects of platelets — diagnosed by platelet function tests.
- Circulating damaged platelets which have been activated and lost their functional capacity — the most common example is the platelet defect following cardiac bypass surgery.

1.6 Thrombocytosis

Platelet counts may rise as high as 2000×10^9/l due to primary myeloproliferation or secondary to causes such as chronic haemorrhage, malignancy, surgery, or inflammatory disorders. In myeloproliferation the spleen may be palpable, but the distinction between the two categories is not always easy to make.

- Small vessel occlusion may cause peripheral ischaemia with bounding pulses, a condition often corrected by antiplatelet drugs.
- Transient ischaemic attacks and large vessel occlusion may also occur.
- Haemorrhage is sometimes seen with very high platelet counts and platelet functional defects may then be demonstrated in the laboratory. Improvement in platelet function often follows correction of the count.

1.7 Disorders of coagulation

Abnormalities of haemostasis may cause:

- Haemorrhage.

- Thrombosis and embolism.
- Mixed patterns.

Haemorrhage

The consequences of thrombocytopenia have already been discussed on p. 6. Clotting factor deficiency results in abnormal bleeding whose character and clinical importance depend on which clotting factor is missing and whether the deficiency is complete or partial.

- Spontaneous bleeding from mucous membranes and the gastrointestinal tract is uncommon, even in severe haemophilia, but urinary tract bleeding in this condition does occur, and cerebral haemorrhage, though rare, is well described.
- Bleeding into joints and muscles is often regarded as 'spontaneous', but each bleed probably follows minor trauma to a moving part.

Following injury, haemorrhage is typically delayed because of the greater importance of the platelets in primary haemostasis. Bleeding is rarely catastrophic initially, and the blood does clot slowly. The result is that large ineffective clots form which either break off from a surface wound to reveal fresh bleeding beneath or track through tissues with the formation of massive haematomas. Problems with tonsillectomy, dental extraction or other surgery, the need for blood transfusions, and the presence of a family history are all very useful pointers to a diagnosis before laboratory tests are undertaken.

Thrombosis

Thrombosis is much more common than abnormal haemorrhage and yet far less is understood about its aetiology. Important risk factors include:

- Age.
- Malignancy.
- Smoking.
- Diabetes mellitus.
- Hyperlipidaemia.

- Hypertension.
- Pregnancy.
- The contraceptive pill.
- Polycythaemia.

Mixed patterns

When the balance between haemostatic activation and its control is disturbed, a syndrome of thrombosis complicated by abnormal bleeding may develop.

- Ischaemic damage may be caused to vital organs, such as the brain and kidneys.
- Clotting factors and platelets are consumed and red cells are injured by passage through a fibrin meshwork leading to microangiopathic haemolytic anaemia (MAHA).
- The fibrinolytic mechanism is activated.

Principal clinical findings include:

- Hypotension.
- Cyanosis.
- Coma and/or focal neurological damage.
- Renal failure and electrolyte disturbances.
- Anaemia.
- Purpura.
- Bruising.
- Haemorrhage from venepuncture sites.

The generic term 'diffuse intravascular coagulation (DIC)' is often applied to this condition, which has a grave prognosis.

2 Systemic manifestations of haematological diseases

2 Systemic manifestations of haematological diseases

Disorders of the blood and the reticuloendothelial system affect many other body systems. In this section each system is dealt with in turn, in the order that they may be encountered during clinical examination of the patient. Many of the presenting features are caused by conditions that are much more common than the haematological problems under discussion.

2.1 Dermatology

A thorough examination of all skin surfaces, including mouth, nails and genitalia, should accompany the normal history and examination.

Common clinical findings

Itching may be localized, generalized, persistent or intermittent. Itching of sudden onset without skin lesions may be seen in lymphomas, especially Hodgkin's disease. Itching related to bathing is often associated with polycythaemia rubra vera.

Ichthyosis is dryness of the skin with thickening and scaling, which may occur when there is an underlying tumour.

Bruising and petechiae may be spontaneous or traumatic and are generally out of proportion to the degree of trauma when associated with thrombocytopenia. Non-thrombocytopenic forms are considered on p. 7.

Telangiectases are localized dilations of venules affecting skin, nasal and oral mucosa, the gastrointestinal tract, the lungs and urinary tract. They are seen in hereditary haemorrhagic telangiectasia.

Nails. Any serious illness may cause slowing of nail growth with a transverse depression across each nail bed.

- Koilonychia describes spoon-shaped nails characteristic of iron-deficiency anaemia.

2 Systemic manifestations of haematological diseases

2.1 Dermatology

- Nail dystrophy occurs in dyskeratosis congenita.

Skin colour:

- Local pigmentation is seen after radiotherapy, while generalized pigmentation may occur in malignant diseases or as a result of cytotoxic drugs, especially busulphan.
- Jaundice is usually slight in haemolytic anaemia and intense jaundice in adults is usually due to obstruction of the biliary system.
- Cyanosis is due to the presence of reduced haemoglobin in the dermal blood vessels.
- Methaemoglobinaemia may mimic the cyanosis of cardiac and pulmonary disease and may be hereditary or secondary to the ingestion of drugs or chemicals.

Exfoliation. Generalized erythema and subsequent shedding of the skin may be accompanied by severe pruritus and systemic upset. Lymphomas of a generalized or cutaneous type are associated with exfoliation but primary skin disease and drug toxicity are commoner causes.

Ulceration is seen on the lower extremities in any chronic haemolytic anaemia, especially sickle cell disease and thalassaemia major. This is often medial, in contrast to that secondary to vascular disease, which tends to be lateral.

- Pyoderma gangrenosum is rarely associated with acute leukaemia.
- Pseudomonas septicaemia, which is common in the immunosuppressed patient, can present with typical lesions which have a dark erythematous surround and a black necrotic centre. The diagnosis may be suspected on these appearances alone.
- Cytotoxic-induced ulceration due to extravasation of drugs causes deep, painful, and poorly healing ulcers. These are especially common when small, peripheral veins are used, and the back of the hand is a particularly vulnerable site.

2.1 Dermatology

Infiltration

Leukaemic infiltrates are usually associated with the monocytic leukaemias.

- Lymphomatous infiltration is rare and may be heralded by non-specific features of itching and dryness.
- Mycosis fungoides primarily affects the dermis and presents as painless, erythematous plaques. On biopsy they show the specific features of pseudo-abscess formation (Pautrier's micro-abscesses).

Drug effects

Many of the drugs used to treat and support patients with haematological disease cause skin problems.

- Alopecia — cytotoxic drugs.
- Photosensitivity rashes — fluorouracil and chlorpromazine.
- Contact dermatitis — many antibiotics, cytotoxics and phenothiazines.
- Erythematous, maculopapular skin eruptions — allopurinol and some antibiotics, especially penicillin and sulphonamides.
- Pigmentation — busulphan.
- Ulceration.

Graft versus host disease (GVHD)

GVHD commonly follows bone marrow transplantation but may occur in any immunosuppressed patient. The name refers to the attack by donor lymphocytes on recipient tissue.

- Acute GVHD affects the gastrointestinal tract and liver but skin lesions are the earliest manifestation. There is a widespread rash, particularly affecting the palms and soles, which is maculopapular, itchy and often scaly. It may progress to erythroderma.
- Chronic GVHD causes 'lichenoid' rash, and frequently a scleroderma-like condition evolves.

2.2 Oral medicine

The mouth is a particularly vulnerable area as it is constantly subject to trauma and has a large resident population of bacteria.

Common clinical findings

Mucosal atrophy is seen in deficiency states due to failure to maintain the rapid turnover of the mucous membrane. In vitamin B_{12} and iron-deficiency anaemia the tongue may be red and smooth and there may be an associated angular stomatitis.

Gingival swelling and superficial ulceration with marked hyperplasia of the gingivae are particularly common in acute and chronic forms of monocytic leukaemia.

Tonsillar enlargement, often unilateral, may be seen in lymphoma. There is usually associated lymph node enlargement.

Necrosis with extensive ulceration of the gingivae, buccal mucosa palate, tonsils and pharynx occurs associated with agranulocytosis of any cause. Methotrexate causes a severe necrotic mucositis.

Infection may occur in any ulcerated area.

- Moniliasis gives rise to creamy white patches. It particularly affects immunosuppressed patients who are being treated with broad-spectrum antibiotics.
- Herpes simplex causes vesicular lesions.

Petechiae, ecchymosis and bleeding gingivae are seen in thrombocytopenia.

- A distressing mixture of necrosis and ulceration, superadded infection and bleeding is commonly seen together in immunosuppressed patients.

2.3 Respiratory medicine

Common clinical findings

Dyspnoea. Patients with anaemia are often short of breath on exertion, and most of the haematological malignancies are associated with increased susceptibility to respiratory infection.

Haemoptysis. Blood-stained sputum associated with infection is usually purulent. Recurrent blood-stained mucoid sputum raises the possibility of tumour. Lymphomas and leukaemia rarely produce endobronchial deposits, and haemoptysis is often related to thrombocytopenia.

Cyanosis is due to an increased amount of reduced haemoglobin or haemoglobin derivatives in the blood. Impaired pulmonary function is the main cause, but it is also seen when systemic venous blood is shunted into the arterial circulation in heart disease.

- *Pulmonary arteriovenous fistulae* are occasionally seen in hereditary haemorrhagic telangiectasia.
- Central cyanosis occurs in hereditary or acquired methaemoglobinaemia.
- In polycythaemia the marked plethora may mimic cyanosis.

Mediastinal obstruction

This may be caused by an enlarged thymus or by mediastinal lymph nodes.

- T-cell acute lymphoblastic leukaemia, which is most common in teenage boys, may present with symptoms of mediastinal obstruction, and this may antedate the development of a leukaemic phase of several weeks. This condition has also been called Sternberg's sarcoma.

Diffuse pulmonary shadows

Diffuse pulmonary shadows on radiography are a common diagnostic problem. When due to lymphoma or leukaemia the diagnosis is usually suggested by general examination and the peripheral blood picture. Hodgkin's disease may, however, arise in and be confined to the lung parenchyma.

Opportunistic infection is an important cause of diffuse pulmonary shadowing in immunosuppressed patients. Implicated agents include:

- *Pneumocystis carinii.*
- Candida and Aspergillus species.
- Cytomegalovirus.
- Herpes zoster and simplex.
- Measles virus.
- Tuberculosis.

Numerous cytotoxic agents may cause lung shadowing secondary to interstitial fibrosis, of which busulphan , bleomycin, methotrexate and melphalan are the most important examples.

Pulmonary eosinophilia, from whatever cause, is usually associated with a blood eosinophilia. The shadows on the chest X-ray tend to be transient.

2.4 Cardiovascular disease

Common clinical findings

Pain. Anaemia imposes increased demands upon the heart and in pre-existing coronary artery disease may provoke angina pectoris or intermittent claudication. When anaemia is severe either pain may be present at rest.

Heart failure. Congestive cardiac failure can be exacerbated or provoked by anaemia.

2.4 Cardiovascular disease

- The dyspnoea, tachycardia and peripheral oedema that occur in severe anaemia may mimic heart disease.
- In idiopathic haemochromatosis and transfusion-dependent anaemia, iron overload causes tissue damage. Fatal arrhythmias and refractory cardiac failure may develop.
- In hypereosinophilic syndromes the ventricular walls may become fibrotic and replaced by dense masses of eosinophilic tissue, resulting in congestive cardiac failure.
- Daunorubicin and adriamycin, used widely to treat leukaemias and lymphomas, are cardiotoxic and cause an irreversible cardiomyopathy that is usually dose-related. Congestive failure may be preceded by electrocardiographic changes but is usually abrupt and often fatal.

Murmurs. Cardiac output may be greatly increased in anaemia leading to an aortic flow murmur.

Cardiac enlargement is a feature of congestive cardiac failure and of pericardial effusion which may be found in lymphoma due to pericardial deposits.

Lymphoma causing mediastinal enlargement may mimic the appearances of cardiac enlargement on X-ray, but there are usually no features of heart disease and conventional or computerized axial tomography may be needed to differentiate the two.

Hypertension. Marked elevation of the systolic pressure alone may be found in patients with high cardiac output due to anaemia or the presence of arteriovenous fistulae. This does not have the same clinical significance as hypertension in which the diastolic pressure is also raised.

Polycythaemia is associated with hypertension, possibly because of the raised intravascular volume and hyperviscosity; this may be seen in some types of myeloma and macroglobulinaemia.

Peripheral vascular disease. In polycythaemia, thrombotic and embolic events are common presenting features. Where there is pre-existing vascular disease the effect may be enhanced, with ulceration, pain and gangrene of the digits, particularly if there is thrombocytosis.

2.5 Gastroenterology

The mouth and anus are particularly vulnerable to injury.

Common clinical findings

Nausea and vomiting are caused by:

- Many of the cytotoxic agents used in the treatment of haematological malignancy.
- Gastric atrophy associated with pernicious anaemia.

There is a small but definite association between blood group A and an increased incidence of gastric carcinoma.

Dysphagia is rarely associated with the formation of a post-cricoid web. A sleeve of increased resistance in the proximal oesophagus or a sheet of mucosa partially occludes the lumen and is associated with severe iron deficiency in the Plummer–Vinson syndrome, leading to an increased incidence of carcinoma of the oesophagus.

- Candidal oesophagitis is an important cause of dysphagia in the severely ill patient, and oral thrush is the most reliable clue to diagnosis.

Haematemesis and melaena is encountered in leukaemia, thrombocytopenia and haemophilia. Lymphomas of the stomach may present with bleeding and a palpable epigastric mass. Polycythaemia rubra vera is associated with an increased incidence of peptic ulceration but may also cause mesenteric and portal vein thrombosis with secondary variceal bleeding due to portal hypertension.

Haemochromatosis may be complicated by haematemesis due to cirrhosis and portal hypertension.

Constipation is a common side-effect of the vinca alkaloids. It is also very common in all patients admitted to hospital and can contribute to perianal infection in susceptible patients if large, hard stools are passed intermittently.

Diarrhoea. Loose stools are a common feature of haematological disease.

- Blood loss may be seen in patients with thrombocytopenia or hereditary telangiectasia, but this is comparatively uncommon in congenital clotting disorders.
- Damage to the bowel wall occurs following radiotherapy, chemotherapy, or immunosuppression in patients with acute leukaemia or aplasia, and infection, including cryptosporidium, is also an important cause of diarrhoea in this group.
- Where broad-spectrum antibiotics have been used, diarrhoea may be severe, especially in the pseudomembranous colitis which is due to *Clostridium difficile*.
- Lymphomatous infiltration of the bowel may lead to protein-losing enteropathy.
- Pernicious anaemia or other causes of vitamin B_{12} deficiency leads to a failure of mucosal development and diarrhoea may result.

Malabsorption

Radiation therapy and cytotoxic agents, by destroying rapidly dividing cells, may predispose to malabsorption. Small bowel lymphoma is a very rare cause of malabsorption, but there is an increased incidence of neoplasia, and in particular lymphoma, of the small intestine in coeliac disease. Congenital or acquired hypogammaglobulinaemia may be a cause of malabsorption.

Ano-rectal abscesses

These are common in immuncompromised patients and may be caused by examination of the anus or by abrasion by hard stool. The infection starts in an anal gland but may spread locally into the ischio-rectal fossa and perianal region or systemically. The anus should be inspected and swabbed regularly but, while the white cell count and platelet count are low, internal examination should be kept to a minimum. As the patient with a low cell count is unable to form pus, local signs of inflammation are not always evident and the first symptoms may be due to systemic illness. Common infective agents include:

- *Escherichia coli*.
- *Staphylococcus aureus*.
- Bacteroides species.

2.6 The liver

The commonest symptom, apart from those discussed in Section 2.5 above, is jaundice, but this may also be due to problems occurring outside the liver itself.

Haemolytic jaundice

Most bilirubin derives from the haemoglobin of degenerating red blood cells, and mild jaundice may occur in any condition with increased red cell breakdown. The blood contains only unconjugated bilirubin, the stools are normal in colour and the urine contains excess urobilinogen which darkens on standing. There is no bilirubin in the urine.

- Haemolytic disease of the newborn may be associated with very high levels of unconjugated bilirubin and there is a risk of kernicterus when the level reaches 340 μmol/l.
- After prolonged haemolysis, pigment gall stones may form and cause obstructive jaundice.

Liver cell jaundice

This is usually due to a mixture of liver cell damage and intrahepatic cholestasis. Infection is the most important cause and may be due to viral hepatitis A, which is spread by the faecal–oral route, or to serum hepatitis (B or non-A, non-B) which is spread by blood or blood products. Other causes of viral hepatitis include:

- Glandular fever.

- Cytomegalovirus.
- Herpes simplex.

Septicaemia may also be associated with acute liver damage and jaundice.

Obstructive jaundice

Pigment gall stones may cause jaundice as the first sign of a previously unrecognized chronic haemolytic process with hyperbilirubinaemia, e.g. hereditary spherocytosis. Patients with established symptomatic haemolysis, e.g. sickle cell disease, may develop superimposed obstructive jaundice from the same cause. Enlarged lymph nodes in the porta hepatis may cause jaundice in the lymphomas.

Drugs

The number of drugs capable of causing jaundice is very great and many different mechanisms are involved.

Haemolysis

- Methyldopa causes autoimmune haemolytic anaemia with a positive direct antiglobulin test (the test is often positive without evidence of haemolysis).
- The 8-aminoquinolones (and others) cause haemolysis in patients with glucose-6-phosphate dehydrogenase (G6PD) deficiency.

Hepatotoxicity

- Anabolic and androgenic steroids, methotrexate, 6-mercaptopurine and thioguanine may cause dose-dependent hepatotoxicity, but individual susceptibility is very variable.
- An acute hepatitis-like syndrome which closely mimics acute viral hepatitis occurs with some antituberculous drugs.

Cholestasis

Chlorpromazine is the most common example, but jaundice is also seen with:

- Antituberculous agents (PAS, rifampicin).
- Other antibiotics (sulphonamides, nitrofurantoin).

There is usually an eosinophilic infiltrate, and occasionally there is a more generalized reaction with fever, a rash, lymphadenopathy and eosinophilia.

Acute liver failure

The most important haematological consequence of this condition is acute haemostatic failure, usually due to a combination of:

- Thrombocytopenia.
- Portal hypertension.
- Failure of coagulation factor synthesis.
- Diffuse intravascular coagulation.

These problems are exacerbated by and contribute to the other features of acute liver failure, especially:

- Encephalopathy.
- Jaundice.
- Renal and electrolyte disorders.
- Sepsis.

The mortality is very high.

2.7 Neurology

Widespread damage may occur to the nervous system as a result of haematological disease. For convenience only, the various aspects are considered on a largely anatomical basis.

The orbit

Lymphomatous deposits occur in the orbit causing unilateral protrusion of the eyeball with exophthalmos, ophthalmoplegia and visual failure.

Retinal haemorrhages are seen in thrombocytopenia, in any form of severe anaemia and also in polycythaemia. Subconjunctival and orbital haemorrhage may also be found in haemophilia.

In the hyperviscosity syndrome associated with the paraproteinaemias, dilated retinal veins with areas of localized narrowing give the appearance of 'sausaging'. There is usually visual impairment, fundal haemorrhages and exudates.

Retinal lesions are seen in sickle cell anaemia and haemoglobin SC disease. Arteriovenous anastomoses occur with peripheral vascular and fibrous proliferation of the retina and areas of black pigmentation. Vitreous haemorrhage and retinal detachment due to fibrous scarring can later lead to blindness. Optic atrophy is a late complication of prolonged and repeated haemorrhage. White leukaemic fundal deposits are often seen in association with haemorrhage.

The nasopharynx

Malignant lymphomas can arise in the nasopharynx presenting with unilateral headache, pain in the trigeminal distribution and cranial nerve palsies.

Skull vault and base

Multiple deposits are seen in myeloma, but these rarely cause symptoms. Lymphomatous deposits cause cranial nerve palsies in some cases.

Intracranial disease

Malignant

Lymphomas may present as primary intracranial tumours; epidural deposits are commoner and cause epileptic seizures with progressive hemiplegia, dysphasia and hemianopia, and are particularly characteristic of the lymphomas complicating immunosuppressive treatment.

Diffuse infiltration is more common in the acute leukaemias, particularly the lymphoid variety. Leukaemic meningitis occurs with headache, neck stiffness, photophobia, vomiting, cranial nerve palsies and clouding of consciousness.

Leptomeningeal infiltration may rarely accompany any focal lymphoma, and when the rest of the CNS is subsequently involved a complex neurological picture can emerge.

2.7 Neurology

Non-malignant complications

Encephalitis or meningitis due to diminished immunity may be bacterial, but yeasts, fungi and viruses, particularly herpes zoster, are very important.

Haemorrhage due to thrombocytopenia occurs and is more frequent when there is bone marrow failure. In haemophilia, intracranial bleeding is rare but is an important cause of death. Cerebral infarction is common in polycythaemia.

Hyperviscosity in the paraproteinaemias causes varying effects on the level of consciousness.

Hypercalcaemia, particularly in myeloma, leads to confusional states.

Leucoencephalopathy due to multifocal demyelination has been described in the lymphoid malignancies.

Spinal disease

- The spine is clinically involved in almost one-third of cases of myeloma, and cord compression occurs in about 6%. Back and root pain are common initial symptoms with progressive paraplegia, sensory loss and sphincter paralysis as spinal cord involvement progresses. The lesion may occur in the vertebral bodies or in the epidural space.
- Neurological complications occur in up to 25% of Hodgkin's disease patients, and more than half are non-metastatic complications. Cord compression is seen in only 4% of patients, the thoracic spine being particularly vulnerable because of the frequency of mediastinal disease.

Peripheral neuropathies

Vitamin B_{12} deficiency may cause a symmetrical 'glove and stocking' neuropathy, the legs usually being affected more than the arms. Paraesthesiae, weakness, difficulty in walking and falling over in the dark are common symptoms. Sensory loss and a positive Romberg sign may be present, reflexes are reduced and the plantar responses are extensor. With severe disease subacute combined degeneration of the spinal cord occurs involving the posterior and lateral columns. As the severity increases and sensory loss in the hands equals that in the legs, spasticity and increased leg reflexes occur. Optic neuropathy and organic dementia are rare.

It is unlikely that folate deficiency causes a similar picture although it often accompanies a variety of chronic neurological disorders.

Tumours can cause direct effects by compression or infiltration of peripheral nerves or roots. Occasionally a non-metastatic neuropathy occurs but the majority of neuropathies in haematological malignancy are due to treatment with the vinca alkaloids.

Clinical evidence of neuropathy is found in more than 10% of patients with myeloma, and in a proportion of these amyloidosis may be found. Similar findings are seen in macroglobulinaemia, cryoglobulinaemia, and polyclonal gammopathies.

Radiotherapy and drug damage

Radiotherapy

Radiation myelopathy produces Lhermitte's sign (paraesthesiae extending down the trunk and limbs when the head is flexed) and may be transient or progressive.

- Cranial irradiation may cause a transient period of somnolence.

Cytotoxic agents

Methotrexate often causes transient meningism with pleocytosis. Meningoencephalopathy can occur several months after discontinuation of a course of treatment, but severe cerebral dysfunction with ataxia and dementia is more often seen following chronic administration. These effects are more pronounced when radiotherapy is given in association with the drug. Seizures and transient paraplegia have also been described.

Procarbazine is a monoamine oxidase inhibitor. It causes disorders of consciousness, ranging from sedation to agitation and psychosis, ataxia and peripheral neuropathy. Manifestations of enzyme inhibition have been described, including orthostatic hypotension, alcohol intolerance, synergism with barbiturates and phenothiazines and sensitivity to catecholamines.

Vincristine may cause seizures and inappropriate ADH secretion but more commonly causes a profound neuropathy affecting the peripheral, cranial and autonomic nerves.

Drug-induced muscle disorders
These are less common than neuropathies, and muscle dysfunction is more likely to be secondary to neuropathy.

- Myasthenic syndromes are described side-effects of aminoglycoside antibiotics, which are commonly used first-line antibiotics in pyrexial immunosuppressed patients.
- Necrotizing myopathies are described with the cytotoxic vinca alkaloids and antifibrinolytic agents. The effect is idiosyncratic and unrelated to dose.
- Painless proximal myopathy is seen with chronic and high-dose corticosteroid therapy.

2.8 Nephrology and urology

Examination of a fresh urine sample is important.

Common clinical findings

Proteinuria
Excretion in excess of 150 mg protein per day is abnormal. The bulk of urinary protein in most renal diseases is albumin, which passes through damaged glomeruli. In myeloma, macroglobulinaemia and primary amyloidosis, the excretion of globulin may exceed albumin and free light chains from the globulin molecule may be found (Bence Jones protein).

2.8 Nephrology and urology

Haematuria

Hereditary or acquired disorders often associated with macroscopic or microscopic bleeding include:

- Anticoagulant therapy.
- Thrombocytopenia — primary or secondary.
- Haemophilia.
- Sickle cell syndromes.

These conditions only account for a small proportion of patients complaining of haematuria, and it should always be remembered that the bleeding disorder may bring to light otherwise unsuspected urinary tract pathology.

Haemoglobinuria

Free haemoglobin is normally bound to carrier proteins and does not appear in the urine unless intravascular haemolysis is gross, saturating the carrier proteins' capacity. To differentiate haemoglobinuria from haematuria, microscopy is useful, as intact red cells will be visible in haematuria. Causes of haemolysis are discussed in Section 4.3. Except for acute exacerbations, many of the chronic hereditary haemolytic anaemias are not associated with haemoglobinuria. Haemosiderinuria following intravascular haemolysis is due to iron deposition in the renal tubules with subsequent shedding into the urine.

Acute renal failure

Pre-renal failure caused by impaired renal perfusion may be due to blood loss or hypotension associated with infection.

Renal failure occasionally occurs following gross intravascular haemolysis, most commonly seen as a result of ABO-incompatible transfusion; otherwise rare it has been described in paroxysmal nocturnal haemoglobinuria (PNH).

Any of the conditions associated with intravascular coagulation may cause intrarenal fibrin to be deposited with rapid deterioration of renal function.

The clinical effects of consumptive coagulopathy are variable:

- Haemolytic uraemic syndrome (HUS): renal failure and microangiopathic haemolytic anaemia (MAHA).
- Thrombotic thrombocytopenic purpura: fever, fluctuating neurological signs, thrombocytopenic purpura, MAHA, and renal failure.
- Septicaemia (usually Gram-negative): diffuse intravascular coagulation (DIC), purpura, renal failure.
- Promyelocytic leukaemia: characteristic morphology of promyelocytes (*see* p. 193) with thrombocytopenia and DIC.

A number of biochemical disturbances may cause or contribute to renal failure:

- Hyperuricaemia may lead to nephropathy and is exacerbated by cytotoxic drugs or radiotherapy. Allopurinol should be given before treatment commences.
- Hypokalaemia develops in many malignant conditions, exacerbating the deterioration of renal function.

Nephrotic syndrome

This syndrome is characterized by severe proteinuria, peripheral oedema, a low plasma protein concentration and an increased blood cholesterol content.

- Renal vein thrombosis has been claimed to cause the nephrotic syndrome, but the thrombotic tendency is sometimes a secondary event, perhaps related to selective loss of antithrombin III in the urine.

Drug-induced disorders of the kidney

Many of the drugs involved in treating haematological disorders may cause renal damage, and as the kidney fails drug accumulation can create a vicious circle.

• Acute nephrotoxicity	Sulphonamides
	Penicillin
	Cephalosporins
	Aninoglycosides
	Amphotericin B

• Interstitial nephropathies	Amphotericin B Antibiotics Mercaptopurine, azathioprine Cyclosporin A
• Crystalluria	Most antimitotic drugs and radiotherapy
• Inappropriate ADH secretion	Sulphonamides Vinca alkaloids Cyclophosphamide
• Haemorrhagic cystitis	Cyclophosphamide Cytosine arabinoside
• Acute tubular necrosis	Methotrexate Doxorubicin

Multiple myeloma and the kidney

Renal failure is commonly associated with myeloma and is a poor prognostic feature. Many of the causative factors are potentially reversible if treatment is commenced early.

- Dehydration.
- Hyperuricaemia.
- Hypercalcaemia.
- Hyperviscosity.
- Infection — both humoral and cellular immunity are impaired and bacterial infection is common.
- Invasion of the kidney by plasma cells.
- Light chain-related tubular damage which may be precipitated by intravenous urography.
- Acquired Fanconi syndrome due to direct damage to the renal tubular epithelium.

Irreversible disease is associated with:

- Amyloidosis, in particular associated with lambda light chains.
- Established renal failure due to the causes listed above.

2.9 Rheumatology and orthopaedics

The painful joint

The differential diagnosis depends on the pattern of joint involvement, associated clinical features and the age of the patient. Acute haemarthrosis is common in severe haemophilia, precipitating trauma often being trivial. Early diagnosis and expert care are important to prevent chronic joint damage.

- Osteomyelitis still occurs in childhood, particularly in sickle cell disease. Typically the infection begins near a joint on the diaphyseal side of the epiphyseal plate and may be accompanied by a 'sympathetic' synovial effusion. Tenderness is maximal beyond the joint line and continues along the bone shaft.
- Gout is an occasional presenting feature in chronic myeloproliferative conditions such as polycythaemia rubra vera, myelofibrosis and chronic granulocytic leukaemia, usually starting in the great toe.
- Avascular necrosis, especially of the hip, may occur in sickle cell syndromes, particularly towards puberty. Similar changes may also be seen in patients on high-dose steroids, possibly due to the osteoporosis induced by these drugs.
- Polyarthritis with effusions, pain and tenderness are not uncommon presentations of childhood acute leukaemia, mimicking juvenile chronic polyarthritis where anaemia and a high white cell count may be seen.
- Henoch–Schönlein purpura is common in childhood and adolescence. There is a characteristic maculopapular eruption with purpura on the buttocks and extensor surfaces of the limbs, associated with an acute migratory arthritis, usually of large joints. Pain is out of proportion to the physical signs. Renal involvement may occur.
- Amyloidosis of the joint capsule mimics rheumatoid arthritis. Bilateral carpal tunnel syndrome may be seen in addition. This type of presentation is usually associated with myeloma.

The painful bone

- Bone pain is a common presenting feature of acute leukaemia, and is a useful pointer to the metamorphosis of chronic granulocytic leukaemia to a more acute phase. Bone marrow necrosis, often associated with leukaemia, causes intense bone pain.

- Myeloma presents with bone pain as a major feature in up to 60% of patients. On X-ray examination osteoporosis is very common, but this condition is also seen in the usual myeloma age group. Sixty to seventy per cent will have discrete bone lesions with a normal alkaline phosphatase level and up to 45% will have hypercalcaemia. Five per cent will suffer a pathological fracture either in the spine or in long bones.
- Sickle cell crisis often presents with generalized bone pain. Localized pain may indicate osteomyelitis.

The painful muscle

Polymyalgia rheumatica presents with proximal muscle pain and stiffness with a raised erythrocyte sedimentation rate. Onset may be acute and symptoms are most severe in the morning.

3 Laboratory investigation and data interpretation

3 Laboratory investigation and data interpretation

3.1 Sampling

The majority of haematological investigations are performed on samples of peripheral venous blood obtained by careful venepuncture with a minimum of occlusion. Free-flowing capillary blood is suitable for preparing a blood film but not for blood counting. Microtechniques requiring much smaller blood samples are often available for paediatric work.

3.1 Sampling

Blood samples are usually taken into the following anticoagulants.

Test	*Anticoagulant*
• Routine haematology	Sequestrene (EDTA)
• ESR	Citrate 1:5
• Viscometry	Sequestrene
• Plasma iron and TIBC	Heparin
• Serum ferritin	Plain glass tube
• Serum B_{12} and folate	Plain glass tube
• Red cell folate	Sequestrene
• Osmotic fragility	Heparin or defibrinated
• Sucrose lysis or Ham's test	Heparin or citrate
• Red cell enzymes	Sequestrene
• Haemoglobin electrophoresis	Sequestrene
• Coagulation and platelet function	Citrate 1:10
• Blood transfusion (Coombs)	Sequestrene
• Blood transfusion (serum)	Plain glass tube
• Haptoglobins	Heparin
• Immunoglobulin studies	Plain glass tube
• Lymphocyte marker studies	Preservative-free heparin

3.2 Interpretation of results

Like all biological measurements the results of haematological tests vary, and this must be taken into account when interpreting any individual result. The three main sources of variation are:

• Methodological — if the same sample is measured a number of times the results will be distributed about a mean. Knowledge of the method used in each laboratory should be known. Now that many laboratories use automated equipment and undertake quality control this variation should be slight.

- Biological — the individual sample from which the result is taken represents one point in time. Factors such as time of day, eating, sleeping, or menstruation may all cause variation. Some tests are very precise and the values vary little within the body. Examples include red cell count, haemoglobin concentration, and mean cell volume, and a change of 10% in these measurements is significant. Others such as the white cell count may vary widely and a change of up to 50% must be persistent before being accepted as abnormal.
- Handling — before accepting unexpected results it is wise to confirm the following:

1 The correct sample has been taken into the correct tube.

2 The correct patient has been bled.

3 The sample has not been left for a prolonged period before testing.

4 Prolonged venous occlusion has not occurred during sampling.

5 There is no evidence of haemolysis or clotting of the sample.

6 The blood has not been taken from an arm which has an infusion running into it.

7 The patient is not taking drugs which will affect the result.

3.3 Basic haematology

The following variables are usually measured:

Haemoglobin concentration (Hb) (g/dl)

Red cell count (RBC) $\times 10^{12}/l$

Mean cell volume (MCV), given in femtolitres (fl)

Haematocrit or packed cell volume (HCT or PCV)

$$= MCV \times RBC$$

Mean cell haemoglobin (MCH) (pg)

$$= \frac{Hb}{RBC}$$

Mean cell haemoglobin concentration (MCHC) (g/dl)

$$= \frac{Hb}{PCV}$$

Anaemia and polycythaemia are defined by the haemoglobin concentration being below or above the normal range for the age and sex of the patient in question, but the number, size and degree of haemoglobinization of the red cells must also be taken into consideration. In practice the most useful measurements are the Hb and MCV in the assessment of anaemia and the Hb and PCV in polycythaemia.

Table 3.1 Normal values for red cell indices.

Age	Hb (g/dl)	MCV (fl)	PCV (%)
1 day	14–22	98–120	50–70
1 year	10–13	70–95	30–40
10 years	11.5–15.5	75–95	35–45
Adult female	12–16	75–99	37–47
Adult male	13–18	75–99	40–54

White cell count (WBC) $\times 10^9$/l

The white cells are counted electronically after lysis of the red cells and the normal range for the total WBC at different ages is shown in Table 3.2.

Table 3.2

Age	Total WBC $\times 10^9$/l
Neonate	10.0–25.0
1 year	6.0–17.0
10 years	4.5–13.5
Adult	4.5–11.0

Platelet count $\times 10^9/l$
Platelets are also counted electronically. The normal range throughout life is 150–450 $\times 10^9/l$.

3.4 The peripheral film

An initial glance with a low-power objective is worthwhile to note agglutination and rouleaux formation as well as to exclude infection with the larger blood parasites but the 'high dry' or oil immersion objective is necessary for detailed study. Each cell type should be considered in turn and abnormalities should be noted.

Red cells

Red cells are non-nucleated biconcave discs approximately 7 μm in diameter and are responsible for oxygen transport. They have an average life-span of 120 days and rely on glycolysis for their metabolism. They do not possess mitochondria and there is no Krebs cycle. Red cell abnormalities are usually due to one of the following:
- Red cell membrane defects.
- Red cell enzyme defects.
- Prolems with haemoglobin synthesis.
- External factors including physical or chemical agents and autoimmune phenomena.

There are numerous descriptive terms applied to the features of red cells in stained films.

Normocytosis. Normal red cells showing the typical biconcave disc shape.

Anisocytosis. Red cells which vary in size to an abnormal degree. This is essentially a subjective assessment although some modern counters do give a measure of red cell distribution width (RDW).

Poikilocytosis. Red cells which may vary in shape to an abnormal degree. Typical descriptions include:

- Teardrop cells — often seen in marrow infiltration.
- Pencil cells — typical of iron deficiency.
- Target cells — seen in iron deficiency, thalassaemia minor and other haemoglobinopathies, in liver disease and after splenectomy.
- Helmet cells, burr cells, acanthocytes, crenated cells, schistocytes and fragmented cells. Classically seen in microangiopathic haemolytic anaemia, uraemia and diffuse intravascular coagulation, and in some inherited conditions.
- Elliptocytes — seen in hereditary elliptocytosis and iron deficiency.
- Spherocytes — small, dense, spherical cells which have lost membrane and are found in hereditary spherocytosis, autoimmune haemolytic anaemia and following physical damage to the red cells.
- Sickle cells — found in sickle cell disease.

Macrocytosis. Cells which are larger than normal and are usually found in deficiencies of vitamin B_{12} or folic acid. Conditions in which macrocytosis may occur, often in association with a normoblastic marrow, include:

- Reticulocytosis due to acute blood loss and haemolytic anaemia.
- Newborn children.
- Leukaemia and pre-leukaemic syndromes.
- Sideroblastic anaemia.
- Myxoedema and hypopituitarism.
- Alcohol abuse.
- Liver disease.
- Bone marrow infiltration.
- Patients who have received certain cytotoxic drugs which interfere with nucleic acid synthesis.

Hypochromia, in which red cells which contain less haemoglobin than normal resulting in a pale colour, and *microcytosis*, in which cells are smaller than normal, usually occur together, and causes include:

- Iron deficiency.

- Thalassaemia.
- Sideroblastic anaemia.
- Anaemia of chronic disease (usually mild).

Polychromasia. Red cells which are purplish in colour when stained with Romanowsky stains owing to the presence of residual ribonucleic acid (RNA) in their cytoplasm. These are young cells and are an index of erythropoiesis. They usually make up less than 2% of peripheral blood red cells. A true increase in reticulocyte numbers typically occurs with haemolysis or haemorrhage, whereas a reduction is found in hypoplastic anaemias and disorders of red cell maturation.

Normoblastosis. Nucleated red cells are found in the peripheral blood in many forms of severe anaemia and when the bone marrow is infiltrated for any reason.

Red cell inclusions. One of the functions of the spleen is to remove any red cell inclusion bodies.

Howell–Jolly bodies are nuclear remnants and are characteristically seen following splenectomy, in megaloblastic anaemia, and in the functional asplenism of sickle cell disease.

Sideroblastic granules are non-haemoglobin iron-containing inclusions giving a positive Prussian blue reaction. They are particularly common in sideroblastic anaemia and following splenectomy, and may also be seen in the newborn.

Punctate basophilic granules are seen in lead poisoning, megaloblastic anaemia and toxic states.

Malarial parasites may be difficult to detect when infestation is light and a prolonged search of thin and thick films may be necessary.

Heinz bodies may be seen after supravital staining with brilliant cresyl blue. They indicate potential red cell instability and are seen in some red cell enzyme deficiencies and haemoglobinopathies following splenectomy.

H bodies are found in haemoglobin H disease, a form of α-thalassaemia, and are also demonstrated by supravital staining. The red cell inclusions are seen as widely distributed stippling.

Rouleaux

Rouleaux formation is a non-specific phenomenon in which red cells, when allowed to settle, lie face to face like piles of coins. It may be prominent when large molecular weight colloids such as fibrinogen and globulins are increased or dextrans are present in the blood, and reduced in polycythaemia, when the high red cell concentration keeps the cells in suspension. Rouleaux can cause difficulty during grouping and cross-matching procedures.

Causes of anaemia

Blood loss	Acute Chronic
Deficiency states	Iron deficiency Vitamin B_{12} deficiency Folic acid deficiency
Haemolysis	Membrane defects Haemoglobin synthetic defects Enzyme defects Extrinsic red cell damage
Bone marrow failure	Aplastic anaemia Infiltration Sideroblastic anaemia
Anaemia of chronic disease	

Blood loss

Following an acute haemorrhage it takes some hours for the haemoglobin concentration to fall. Initially there is a normocytic normochromic anaemia with leucocytosis and thrombocytosis, but as the bone marrow is stimulated by the blood loss polychromatic macrocytes appear and nucleated red cells may be seen in severe cases. Finally, if iron stores are exhausted a hypochromic microcytic anaemia may follow.

Deficiency states

Iron deficiency. A lack of iron for haemoglobin synthesis results in a hypochromic microcytic anaemia with marked anisocytosis, poikilocytosis and target cell formation.

Macrocytic anaemia. The most important cause of macrocytosis is megaloblastic anaemia due to a deficiency of vitamin B_{12} or folic acid. In severe cases megaloblastic nucleated red cells may appear in the peripheral blood. In addition, white cell and platelet production is abnormal, causing leucopenia with hypersegmented neutrophils and thrombocytopenia. Acute blood loss or any form of haemolysis may cause macrocytosis and polychromasia because of the release of young red cells into the circulation.

Haemolysis

Red cell destruction may be extravascular, when red cells are removed by the spleen, or intravascular, when haemoglobin may appear in the urine. Mixed patterns also occur.

The peripheral film often shows polychromasia and macrocytosis and nucleated red cells may be released into the peripheral blood. The biochemical consequences of haemolysis are discussed on p. 64. Specific red cell changes depend on the cause of haemolysis:

Hereditary spherocytosis	microspherocytes
Hereditary elliptocytosis	elliptocytes
Thalassaemias	hypochromia and microcytosis
Sickle cell disease	sickle cells
Enzyme deficiencies	normocytosis
Autoimmune haemolysis (warm)	microspherocytes
(cold)	agglutination
Physical damage	red cell fragmentation

Bone marrow failure

Aplastic anaemia. A failure of bone marrow stem cells usually leads to a normocytic normochromic anaemia, usually accompanied by leucopenia and thrombocytopenia.

Infiltration. When the bone marrow is infiltrated by primary or secondary neoplasm, fibrous tissue, bone or storage disorder cells, the bone marrow release mechanism breaks down and immature white cells and nucleated red cells appear in the peripheral blood. This is called leucoerythroblastic anaemia.

Sideroblastic anaemia. There is a failure to incorporate iron into haem. This may be primary or secondary to a variety of disease states (*see* p. 134).

The effect on red cell morphology is variable, and either microcytosis or macrocytosis may occur.

Anaemia of chronic disease
Anaemia is likely to complicate any long-standing inflammatory or malignant condition. The anaemia of chronic disease is typically normocytic and normochromic, but some hypochromia and microcytosis may occur. The principal defects are a failure to transfer iron from the reticuloendothelial system to the erythroblasts together with a shortened red cell survival.

Table 3.3 Some common examples of anaemia.

	Normal	Iron deficiency	Thalassaemia minor	Anaemia of chronic disease	Macrocytic anaemia
Hb	14.7	6.7	10.7	10.6	5.3
RBC	5.0	4.1	5.4	3.5	1.4
MCV	84	59	60	91	113
PCV	42	25	32	33	16
MCH	30	16	20	30	36
MCHC	35	27	30	32	32

Polycythaemia

The red cells are usually normal morphologically, whatever the cause, unless the patient has become iron deficient through expansion of the red cell mass or by venesection or haemorrhage. Elevation of the white cell count and platelet count are useful pointers to polycythaemia rubra vera, and in the later stages of this condition myelofibrosis may lead to leucoerythroblastic anaemia, or acute leukaemia may develop.

Table 3.4 Polycythaemia.

	Normal	Secondary polycythaemia	Polycythaemia vera (PRV)	PRV with iron deficiency
Hb	14.7	21	21	18.5
RBC	5.0	7.2	7.2	8.4
MCV	84	93	93	68
PCV	42	67	67	56
MCH	30	30	30	22
MCHC	35	32	32	31
WBC	7.0	5.0	14.5	12.0
Platelets	300	200	540	600

White cells

Most white cells are 10–15 μm in diameter although some lymphocytes are rather smaller than this.

Granulocytes and monocytes are involved in the acute inflammatory response.

Lymphocytes are involved in the immune response, in conjunction with monocytes.

Table 3.5 Typical differential white cell counts.

Age	Total count $\times 10^9/l$	Granulocytes (%) Neutrophils	Eosinophils	Basophils	Monocytes	Lymphocytes
1 year	6.0–17.0	30	3	<1	5	62
10 years	4.5–13.5	55	3	<1	4	38
Adult	4.5–11.0	60	3	<1	4	33

Granulocytes

These cells are divided into three groups depending on the staining characteristics of their granules.

Neutrophils have polymorphic nuclei, usually with three or four lobes, and contain two main types of granule:

- Azurophilic or primary granules containing myeloperoxidase.
- Specific or secondary granules containing lysozyme, alkaline phosphatase, lactoferrin, and B_{12} binding protein. It is these granules which stain neutrally with Romanowsky dyes.

The bone marrow takes up to 14 days to produce a neutrophil, but these cells only remain in the circulation for a few hours before entering the tissues by a process called margination. Granulocytes have irreversibly lost the ability to divide and synthesize new cellular protein. Their function is to combat infection and injury by the following properties.

- Mobility.
- Chemotaxis.

- Phagocytosis.
- Bacterial killing.

The following morphological changes are recognized:

1 During neutrophil activity granulation is often enhanced and is known as 'toxic granulation'.

2 Light blue cytoplasmic inclusions called Döhle bodies are sometimes seen in toxic states. These are also seen in the May–Hegglin anomaly.

3 In the congenital Chédiak–Higashi syndrome the neutrophils contain giant eosinophilic granules.

4 Reduced secondary granulation is characteristic of chronic granulocytic leukaemia (CGL) but may also occur in other myeloid leukaemias.

5 The Pelger–Huët anomaly is a congenital condition in which neutrophil lobulation is reduced. The effects of infection, leukaemia, and drugs may also produce an acquired form of this phenomenon.

6 When immature neutrophils appear in the peripheral blood, with a reduction or absence of nuclear lobulation, this is called a 'left shift'. It is usually due to increased white cell release in response to inflammation or injury.

7 When there is excessive nuclear lobulation the term 'right shift' is used. There is an increase from the normal four to five lobes to six or more in a majority of cells. It is found in:

- Megaloblastic anaemia.
- Renal failure.
- Iron deficiency.
- Hereditary neutrophil hypersegmentation.

Neutrophil leucocytosis occurs in response to almost any stimulus due to the large storage pool in the bone marrow which can be mobilized rapidly in response to any insult. Causes of a neutrophilia are discussed in more detail in Section 4.4.

Neutropenia signifies a reduction in the neutrophil count below the normal range. Once the count has fallen below 1.0×10^9/l the risk of infection increases. The count may be low because of a congenital hereditary defect or there may be an acquired cause. A neutrophil count which would be low in a Caucasian population may be physiological in Africans and West Indians and is not associated with any clinical abnormality. The acquired causes are in general more clinically important and may be due to defective granulopoiesis, removal from the circulation or in relation to intercurrent infection and are considered in more detail in Section 4.4.

Neutrophil dysfunction. Some patients, while having normal neutrophil numbers, are still prone to infection. This may be due to a congenital or acquired functional abnormality.

Alteration in ability to destroy bacteria	Chronic granulomatous disease Chédiak–Higashi syndrome Myeloperoxidase deficiency Leukaemia
Impaired complement function	Impaired chemotaxis Lazy leucocyte syndrome
Impaired phagocytosis and motility	Diabetes mellitus Uraemia Paraproteinaemias Colchicine Ethanol

Eosinophils usually have bilobed nuclei and their cytoplasm is packed with densely staining pink enzymatic granules. An increase is seen in a variety of allergic, parasitic, neoplastic and skin-related disorders (*see* Section 4.4).

Basophils are rarely seen in the normal peripheral blood but are easily recognized by their purplish cytoplasmic granules which obscure the nucleus. The granules contain heparin and histamine and are released during immediate hypersensitivity reactions. These cells are related to tissue mast cells.

Basophilia describes an excess of basophils in the blood and typically occurs in CGL and other myeloproliferative conditions.

Monocytes are large cells with grey–blue cytoplasm, and their nuclei are often kidney-shaped. They are the circulating form of the tissue macrophage and are capable of phagocytosis and pinocytosis. They play a part in the initiation of the immune response by processing antigens but are also involved in the effector arm.

Monocytosis occurs in a variety of inflammatory, infective, and malignant conditions (*see* Section 4.4).

Lymphocytes
These cells are formed in the lymphoreticular system, including the bone marrow. They are divided into two main groups depending on whether they are devoted to cell-mediated immunity (T-cells) or humoral immunity (B-cells), but a distinction between the two types of cells cannot usually be made by simple morphology. A small percentage of cells cannot be identified as B- or T-cells and are known as K or killer cells.

Lymphoid tissue
Bone marrow follicles
Thymus
Lymph nodes
Spleen
Gut-related
  tonsils
  appendix
  Peyer's patches

Differentiation of lymphocytes:

T-cells
: Rosette with unsensitized, washed sheep red cells
: React with antisera raised against T-cells
: Have surface receptors for the Fc portion of IgG and IgM

B-cells
: Possess surface immunoglobulin
: Have surface receptors for the Fc component of immunoglobulin (EA)
: Have receptors for complement components (EAC)
: Rosette with mouse red cells

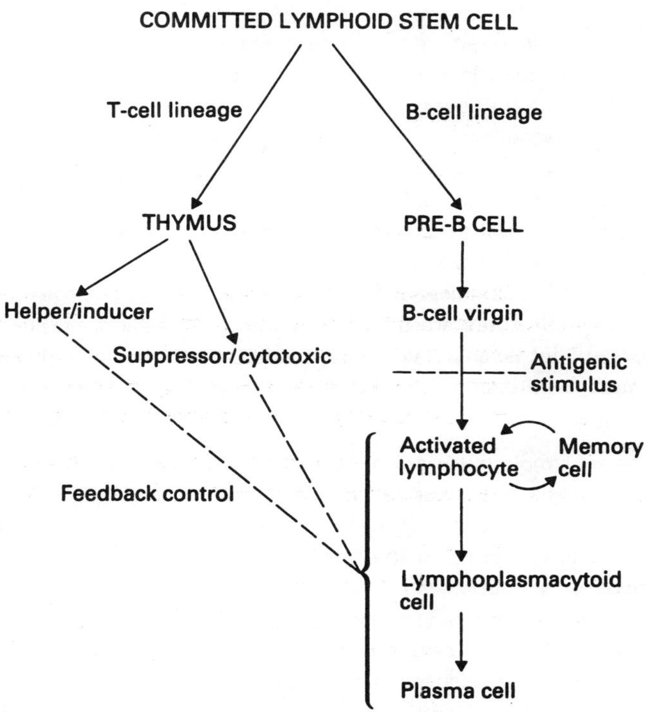

Fig. 3.1 Differentiation of lymphocytes — developmental pathway.

T-cells make up about 40–80% of blood lymphocytes and are 'educated' in the thymus and migrate to T-dependent areas in peripheral lymphoid organs. They play an important role in regulation of the immune response, in graft rejection, delayed hypersensitivity and the activation of macrophages. These functions are achieved by so-called 'helper' and 'suppressor' subsets, which are found in a ratio of approximately 2:1. Specific mouse monoclonal antisera have been used to define which cells belong to the helper/inducer and suppressor/cytotoxic subsets. They also define the various stages in T-cell development.

B-cells are generated in the bone marrow and migrate to the follicular and medullary areas of lymphoid organs. They produce antibodies and are usually recognized by the presence of specific surface or cytoplasmic immunoglobulin. They make up approximately 15–30% of the blood lymphocytes. They contain the heavy chains of IgG, IgM, IgA, or IgD on their surface, occasionally bearing more than one of these. They are however restricted to one light chain type (κ or λ) which are found in a ratio of approximately 2:1. This allows the identification of monoclonality in B-cell malignancy. Resting lymphocytes are usually small and contain only a rim of cytoplasm, but when activated by specific stimuli they enlarge and their cytoplasm becomes deep blue and more conspicuous.

Atypical lymphocytes are particularly characteristic of infectious mononucleosis (glandular fever), cytomegalovirus infections and toxoplasmosis. The atypical cells are T-suppressor cells which are produced in response to the infected B-cells. In the acute early phase of HIV infection, when a glandular fever-like illness may occur, similar atypical lymphocytes appear in the peripheral blood.

Plasma cells are B-cells committed to antibody formation and have an eccentric nucleus with deep-blue cytoplasm and a conspicuous, pale, perinuclear Golgi apparatus. They are rarely seen in the peripheral blood but are common in the bone marrow and in lymph nodes. As each lymphocyte has a specific potential, the distinction between neoplastic and inflammatory lymphocyte disorders can be made by looking for evidence of monoclonal, as opposed to polyclonal, proliferation, and this is a useful diagnostic tool.

Malignant change can be assumed if the cells involved can be demonstrated to be monoclonal in nature.

Lymphopenia is associated with:

- Congenital immunodeficiency syndromes (*see below*) and a variety of disease states which are discussed later (Section 4.4) particularly associated with DXT and drug administration.

Congenital disorders of lymphocyte function:

Bursa-dependent	Primary immunoglobulin deficiency X-linked congenital agammaglobulinaemia (Bruton) Dysgammaglobulinaemia IgA deficiency
Thymus-dependent	Thymic dysplasia with normal immunoglobulins (Nezelof) Thymic aplasia and parathyroid deficiency (Di George)
Combined immune deficiency	Reticular dysgenesis (also affects granulocytes) Swiss-type agammaglobulinaemia (SCID) Hereditary ataxia telangiectasia

Platelets

Platelets are small granular discoid bodies approximately 2–4 μm in diameter and are composed of fragments of megakaryocyte cytoplasm. Their essential functions of adhesion, aggregation, nucleotide release and clot retraction are considered in more detail in the section on the laboratory investigation of haemostatic disorders (p. 88) but much can be learned by studying their appearance in stained films. The most important features are platelet size and platelet numbers. Occasionally platelet clumping also occurs, despite careful sample preparation, due to the EDTA anticoagulant, but this problem can usually be overcome by taking the blood into citrate. Clumping is obvious if blood is spread directly from a finger prick.

Platelet size

Small platelets are characteristic of the Wiskott–Aldrich syndrome. Large platelets occur in:

- Thrombocytopenia due to platelet loss or destruction.
- Myeloproliferative disease.
- Patients following splenectomy.
- The May–Hegglin anomaly.
- Bernard–Soulier disease.

Thrombocytopenia has many causes, but most examples fall into one of the following categories:

1 *Failure of production due to*:

- Aplasia.
- Bone marrow infiltration.
- Deficiency of vitamin B_{12} or folic acid.
- Congenital causes.

2 *Dilution* following:

- Massive transfusion of stored blood.

3 *Destruction and/or pooling* in:

- Isoimmune or autoimmune states.
- Hypersplenism.
- Diffuse intravascular coagulation (DIC).
- Thrombotic thrombocytopenic purpura (TTP).

Thrombocytosis usually occurs as a primary phenomenon in myeloproliferative disorders such as polycythaemia rubra vera, chronic granulocytic leukaemia and essential thrombocythaemia. There are also many secondary causes of an elevated platelet count usually related to inflammation in its widest sense:

- Injury and surgery.
- Infection.
- Rheumatoid arthritis.
- Inflammatory bowel disease.
- Chronic haemorrhage.
- Hodgkin's disease.
- Other malignancy.
- Splenectomy.
- Post-natal.

Post-splenectomy

Removal of the spleen produces characteristic changes in the peripheral blood.

Red cells

- Anisocytosis.
- Target cells.
- Howell–Jolly bodies.
- Siderocytes.

White cells

- Leucocytosis with a 'left shift'.

Platelets

- Thrombocytosis which may reach 1000×10^9/l and is sometimes persistent.

3.5 Erythrocyte sedimentation rate (ESR)

For many years the rate of sedimentation of red cells in whole blood has been used as a non-specific index of disease. The rate of sedimentation depends on the haematocrit and the protein concentration of the plasma, particularly fibrinogen and globulin. Quoted normal values are up to 5 mm for men and up to 10 mm for women but in practice there is little cause for anxiety below 25 mm. The ESR tends to be higher in the elderly even in the absence of disease.

Causes of a high ESR are:

- Infection, inflammation and trauma.
- Malignant disease, especially myelomatosis.
- Collagen vascular disease including temporal arteritis.
- Autoantibodies including cold agglutinin disease.
- Anaemia.

The ESR is reduced in:

- Polycythaemia.

3.6 Haematinic estimation

Iron

Iron is essential for haemoglobin manufacture and is also used in myoglobin, cytochromes and other enzyme systems. It is absorbed from the upper small bowel as ferrous iron but is transported as ferric iron on the glycoprotein transferrin. It may then be reconverted to the ferrous form and used for haemoglobin synthesis or it may be incorporated into the body stores within the bone marrow, liver and spleen. The iron is stored in the ferric form as the soluble protein ferritin, which is detectable in serum, or as the insoluble haemosiderin, which may be stained by the Prussian blue method. Potential routes of iron loss are limited, being confined to haemorrhage and to natural shedding from epithelial surfaces.

Normal values for iron

Total body iron	3–5 g
Haemoglobin iron	2–3 g
Storage iron	1–2 g

3.6 Haematinic estimation

Myoglobin	300–400 mg
Enzyme iron	50–100 mg
Transferrin iron	3–4 mg
Daily oral intake	10 mg or more
Daily absorption	1–2 mg or more
One unit of packed red cells	200 mg
Plasma iron	Men 13–32 μmol/l (70–180 μg/dl) Women 10–30 μmol/l (55–160 μg/dl)
Total iron binding capacity (TIBC)	45–70 μmol/l (250–400 μg/dl)
Serum ferritin	Men 25–400 μg/l Women 15–300 μg/l

Plasma iron (Fe) refers to transferrin-bound iron which is measured colorimetrically.

Latent iron binding capacity (LIBC) is the additional quantity of iron which can be bound to transferrin when iron is added to plasma.

Total iron binding capacity (TIBC) is the sum of the plasma Fe and the LIBC.

Percentage saturation is the ratio of plasma Fe to TIBC expressed as a percentage, and together with the above investigations is valuable in the assessment of iron deficiency, iron overload and the anaemia of chronic disease.

Serum ferritin is found in the circulation in minute quantities and may be measured by radioimmunoassay. Levels below 15 μg/l indicate iron deficiency, but inflammatory conditions may bring the ferritin concentration into the normal range despite the presence of iron deficiency. The serum ferritin is markedly elevated in gross iron overload but intermediate results may be of limited value.

3.6 Haematinic estimation

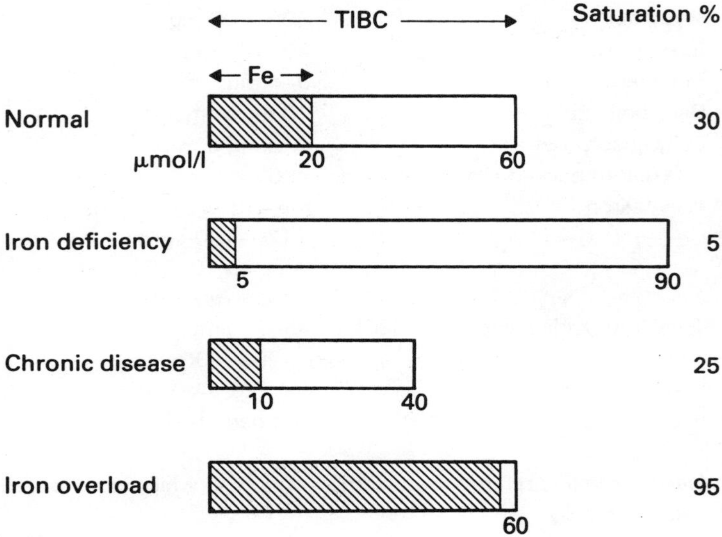

Fig. 3.2 Typical plasma Fe and TIBC values.

Bone marrow iron is easily examined by staining bone marrow aspirates with the Prussian blue method (ferrocyanide). It is really only possible to say whether iron is absent, normal or increased by examining the fragments, but high-power examination of the normoblasts is very helpful in the diagnosis of sideroblastic anaemia.

Liver biopsy specimens can be used to estimate iron overload, and there is the added advantage that liver histology can be assessed at

Table 3.6 Bone marrow iron stores.

	Absent	Normal	Increased
Normal		√	
Iron deficiency	√		
Chronic disease		√	
Iron overload			√

the same time. CT scanning and magnetic resonance imaging may be used to assess body iron in future.

Removal of iron may be used in patients with iron overload to assess iron stores and to treat at the same time.

Vitamin B_{12}

Vitamin B_{12} is a cobalt-containing vitamin or cobalamin which is synthesized by bacteria but is found only in animal products. It plays a vital role in single-carbon transfers and acts as a cofactor for the conversion of:

- Methylmalonic acid to succinic acid.
- Homocysteine to methionine.

The latter reaction is involved in a complex way with folic acid in DNA synthesis, the conversion of

- Deoxyuridine to thymidine.

being one of the principal points of contact in the function of the two vitamins.

Intrinsic factor (IF) is a product of the parietal cells in the gastric antrum and must be linked to vitamin B_{12} before it can be absorbed in the terminal ileum. The vitamin is then transported on the carrier protein transcobalamin II to the liver stores, where there is usually sufficient to last about three years.

Vitamin B_{12} values

Daily requirement	2–5 μg
Body stores	2–3 mg
Serum B_{12}	210–920 ng/l

Deficiency of vitamin B_{12} results in macrocytic megaloblastic anaemia, and more rarely in peripheral neuropathy and subacute combined degeneration of the cord.

Serum B_{12}

A low vitamin B_{12} level usually indicates true deficiency, but low levels are sometimes found in healthy people. Some pregnant women have low levels without having depleted body stores, and this can also occur in patients with folic acid deficiency.

- Children with transcobalamin II deficiency have megaloblastic anaemia with normal vitamin B_{12} levels.

Raised levels of vitamin B_{12} are found in liver disease, myeloproliferative disorders, renal failure, and after B_{12} treatment.

B_{12} absorption tests (Schilling test)

These tests have been designed to analyse the cause of vitamin B_{12} deficiency and to distinguish between a lack of IF and general malabsorption. Radioactive isotopes of cobalt are incorporated into free or IF-bound cobalamin and used to assess absorption of the vitamin. Reduced absorption of vitamin B_{12} alone with correction using the B_{12}/IF combination is usually due to pernicious anaemia. If neither isotope is absorbed then a diagnosis of ileal malabsorption should be considered, but other possible causes include:

- The secretion by a patient with pernicious anaemia of intrinsic factor antibodies into the gastric juice causing neutralization of bound IF.
- Damage to the ileal mucosa by deficiency of vitamin B_{12} which is required for epithelial synthesis as well as haemopoiesis.

For this reason it is often worth delaying B_{12} absorption tests for a few weeks in severe megaloblastic anaemia to allow the bowel

Table 3.7 Vitamin B_{12} absorption tests.

	B_{12} alone	B_{12} + IF
Normal	+	+
Dietary deficiency	+	+
Pernicious anaemia (treated)	−	+
Malabsorption	−	−

+ indicates >10% of the administered dose in a 24-hour urine sample.

mucosa to respond to treatment. Occasionally complete recovery may take longer than this.

Other tests
In pernicious anaemia circulating antibodies are found to:

- Parietal cells in over 90% of patients.
- Intrinsic factor in over 50% of patients.
- The thyroid in 50% of patients.

and gastric acid secretion is markedly reduced or absent.

Folic acid
Folic acid is pteroyl glutamic acid, the pteroyl part of the molecule consisting of a pteridine ring attached to para-amino benzoic acid. Although widely distributed in foodstuffs, vegetables and fruits are a particularly rich source, but folic acid is easily destroyed by prolonged cooking. The vitamin is absorbed throughout the small bowel, is reduced to the tetrahydrofolate form by dihydrofolic acid reductase and circulates as 5-methyltetrahydrofolate. Within the cell glutamic acid residues are added to form polyglutamates, which then act as a coenzyme in the formation of methionine and in nucleic acid synthesis, including the production of thymidine. It is within these pathways that the interaction with vitamin B_{12} takes place so that deficiency of folic acid results in macrocytic megaloblastic anaemia which is morphologically indistinguishable from that due to vitamin B_{12} deficiency. Folic acid deficiency is not usually associated with neurological disease.

Folic acid values

Daily requirement	50–200 μg
Body stores	5–10 mg
Serum folic acid	2–14 μg/l
Red cell folic acid	125–600 μg/l

Folate stores last for about three months in the resting state. Any increase in metabolism is likely to lead to an increased demand for folic acid, as in:

- Pregnancy.
- Haemolytic anaemia.
- Myeloproliferation.
- Neoplastic disease.
- Seriously ill patients in intensive care wards.

Serum folate and red cell folate

A low serum folate is found in:

- Folic acid deficiency.
- Generalized illness.

A high serum folate is found:

- After folate therapy.
- In vitamin B_{12} deficiency.
- After haemolysis of the sample being tested.

Red cell folate levels reflect true body folate status at the time of red cell formation more accurately and a reduced cell folate is good evidence of overall folate deficiency, except in B_{12} deficiency where folate transport across the red cell membrane is impaired.

Deoxyuridine suppression test

This specialized test uses bone marrow to measure the body's ability to convert deoxyuridine to thymidine, a step which is dependent on both vitamin B_{12} and folic acid. Tritium-labelled thymidine is added to the marrow, and in normal circumstances deoxyuridine suppresses radioactive thymidine incorporation into DNA so that less than 10% of the label appears in the nucleic acid. If B_{12} or folic acid is deficient, more labelled thymidine is taken up. If the abnormality is not corrected by vitamin B_{12} addition then this indicates that folic acid was deficient in the original marrow. Deficiency of vitamin B_{12} can be corrected by either B_{12} or folate, and folate can, of course, correct deficiencies of folic acid.

3.7 The diagnosis of haemolysis

Clinical features

Haemolysis causes:

3.7 The diagnosis of haemolysis

- Anaemia.
- Mild jaundice in adults.
- Severe jaundice in neonates.
- Urine which darkens on standing due to the presence of urobilinogen.

In many cases, especially those which are chronic and/or mediated by warm IgG antibodies:

- The spleen is enlarged.

Severe chronic haemolysis due to haemoglobin disorders stimulates haemopoiesis and iron absorption, leading to:

- Expansion of the bone marrow space, especially in the skull (hair on end appearances on X-ray).
- Stunting of growth.
- Damage to the liver, heart and endocrine organs by iron overload.
- Failure of sexual development.

Prolonged haemolytic anaemia can lead to:

- Leg ulceration.
- Pigment gall stones.

If the haemolysis is acute and intravascular there may be:

- Frank haemoglobinuria when the urine appears red or smoky.
- Fever, rigors or loin pain.
- Renal failure.

Simple laboratory tests

Blood

1 The Hb concentration, RBC and PCV are reduced in uncompensated haemolysis.

2 The MCV may be increased as young cells are released from the bone marrow. Microspherocytes, if present, may mask this increase.

3 The MCHC may be increased if microspherocytes are present as they have lost membrane but retained haemoglobin.

4 The white cell count and platelet count may be elevated.

5 The reticulocyte count is usually increased.

6 The peripheral film may show characteristic red cell changes:

- General effects
  - Macrocytosis
  - Polychromasia
  - Normoblastosis
- Specific effects
  - Spherocytosis
    - hereditary
    - autoimmune
    - toxic
  - Elliptocytosis
    - hereditary
  - Sickle cells
    - sickle cell disease
  - Target cells
    - haemoglobin disorders
  - Fragments
    - microangiopathy
  - Burr cells
  - Helmet cells
  - Acanthocytes

7 Unconjugated hyperbilirubinaemia is due to red cell breakdown taking place faster than liver cell conjugation.

8 The effects of free haemoglobin entering the circulation, usually in intravascular haemolysis, are:

- Reduction in haptoglobin — haemoglobin binds to haptoglobin and is removed as a complex by the reticuloendothelial system.
- Methaemalbumin formation — haemoglobin binds to albumin and can be detected spectroscopically.
- Haemoglobinaemia — once the binding properties of the plasma are exhausted free haemoglobin circulates in the plasma and will appear in the urine.

9 Folic acid deficiency may complicate chronic haemolysis.

Urine

1 Excess urobilinogen will be present but *not* bilirubin.

2 Haemoglobinuria occurs when all the plasma binding potential is saturated.
3 Haemosiderin is found in spun urinary deposit following haemoglobinuria. The renal tubules reabsorb the haemoglobin and convert the iron to haemosiderin, which appears in the urine as the tubular cells are shed.

Other tests

Red cell survival
If a haemolytic process is suspected but not proved, red cells can be labelled with radioactive chromium (^{51}Cr) and reinjected. The time taken for half the isotope to disappear ($T_{1/2}$) is normally about 28 days, and a $T_{1/2}$ shorter than 15 days indicates a haemolytic process.

Direct antiglobulin test (*see* p. 81)
This is not a test for haemolysis as such, but should be performed whenever haemolysis is suspected. It is extremely valuable in distinguishing between autoimmune haemolysis (positive result) and other causes (negative result).

3.8 The red cell membrane

Numerous red cell membrane defects exist, but most are diagnosed by the appearance of the peripheral blood film rather than by more elaborate laboratory tests. Two simple groups of tests are also in use for the analysis of these defects.

Red cell osmotic fragility test

The osmotic fragility test assesses the sensitivity of fresh heparinized or defibrinated blood to the hypotonic stimulus of various strengths of buffered saline. Spherocytes, *however caused*, are very sensitive to osmotic stress because of their small membrane surface to cell volume ratio, whereas normal biconcave discs are relatively resistant. Even more resistant are cells which are relatively

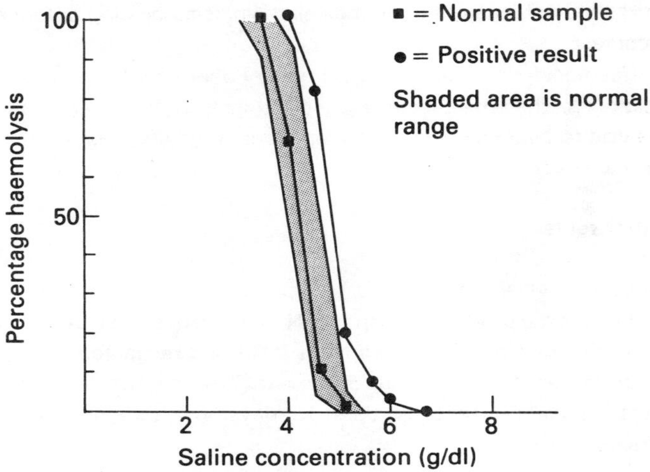

Fig. 3.3 Osmotic fragility test.

overprovided with membrane compared to their haemoglobin content. Increased osmotic fragility is found in:

- Hereditary spherocytosis.
- Autoimmune haemolytic anaemia (especially that due to warm IgG antibodies).
- Toxic red cell damage.

Reduced osmotic fragility is found in:

- Iron deficiency.
- Thalassaemia.
- Sideroblastic anaemia.
- Young red cells (reticulocytes).

To increase the sensitivity of the test the blood can be incubated at 37 °C for 24 hours before testing. The control sample must obviously be treated in the same way.

Tests for paroxysmal nocturnal haemoglobinuria

These tests rely on the non-antibody mediated fixation of complement by the abnormal red cells in paroxysmal nocturnal haemoglobinuria (PNH).

Sucrose lysis test
This uses the increased sensitivity of PNH cells to low ionic strength media.

Acidified serum lysis test (Ham's test)
This test is used to confirm the diagnosis of PNH, but in this case a reduction in pH is used to enhance complement fixation and bring about lysis. A positive result with appropriate negative controls usually means that the patient has PNH.

- In the hereditary dyserythropoietic anaemia (HEMPAS) in which Ham's test is positive, a negative result is obtained using the patient's own acidified serum.
- Negative results may be obtained in transfused patients with PNH.

3.9 Red cell enzymes

Mature red cells lack a nucleus, mitochondria and ribosomes, so that they do not have a tricarboxylic acid cycle and cannot synthesize new protein. They rely entirely on glycolysis to maintain their integrity, and their life-span is limited by the natural decay of enzyme activity within the cell.

ATP is produced by the metabolism of glucose to pyruvate through a number of enzymes, including pyruvate kinase (PK), and within this pathway lies 2, 3-diphosphoglycerate (2, 3-DPG), which helps to control haemoglobin oxygen affinity. NADH is also produced and helps to prevent methaemoglobin formation through methaemoglobin reductase.

Of vital importance to the red cell is the hexose monophosphate shunt, which generates NADPH through glucose-6-phosphate dehydrogenase (G6PD) and 6-phosphogluconate dehydrogenase (6PGD). This NADPH maintains glutathione (GSSG) in the reduced state (GSH), and GSH protects red cell proteins from oxidation.

3.9 Red cell enzymes

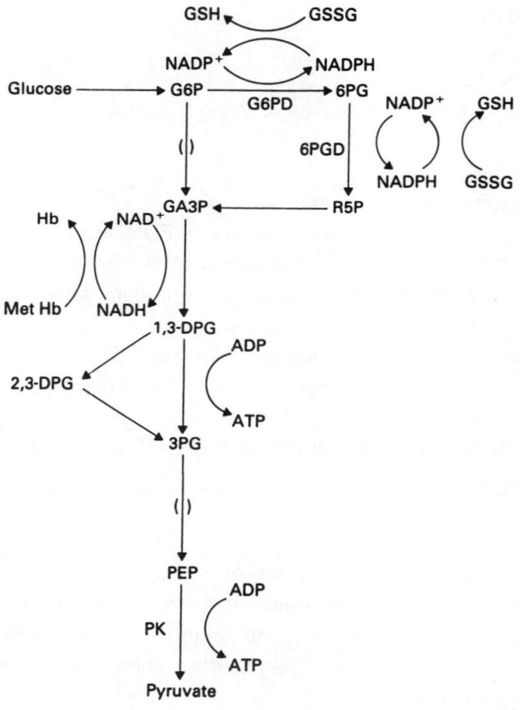

Fig. 3.4 Red cell metabolism of glucose (much simplified).

Key

G6P = Glucose 6-phosphate
GA3P = Glyceraldehyde 3-phosphate
1,3-DPG = 1,3-Diphosphoglycerate
2,3-DPG = 2,3-Diphosphoglycerate
3PG = 3-Phosphoglycerate
PEP = Phosphoenolpyruvate
PK = Pyruvate kinase
G6PD = G6P dehydrogenase
6PG = 6-Phosphogluconate
6PGD = 6PG dehydrogenase
R5P = Ribulose 5-phosphate
GSSG = Glutathione
GSH = Reduced glutathione
Hb = Haemoglobin
Met Hb = Methaemoglobin
(|) indicates summarized pathway

3.9 Red cell enzymes

In practice most physicians will only see patients with G6PD deficiency and PK deficiency, and the former is usually easily diagnosed clinically because it is X-linked and is exacerbated by certain drugs. NADH-mediated methaemoglobin reductase deficiency, when it occurs, is obvious because the patient is cyanosed.

Tests for G6PD deficiency

There are many variants of G6PD found throughout the world, their biological activity varying from normal to zero, and for any given subject young red cells will contain more enzyme than old cells. G6PD deficiency is X-linked. Knowledge of these facts is important in understanding the natural history of G6PD deficiency and in interpreting the results of laboratory tests.

1 Males are more likely to haemolyse than females, but females are not immune. Individual red cells will be either normal or deficient in G6PD depending on which X chromosome was functioning during erythropoiesis.

2 Assay of G6PD during or just after haemolysis may give misleading results as new, comparatively normal, cells are released into the circulation.

3 Because young cells contain greater amounts of G6PD and 6PGD to an equal extent the problem discussed in **2** may be solved by measuring the G6PD/6PGD ratio.

4 Detection of heterozygotes may be made easier by measuring the G6PD/6PGD ratio.

Screening tests for the detection of G6PD deficiency are available and are useful for selecting patients who require further investigation. The most satisfactory technique, however, is the assay of G6PD and 6PGD directly in a spectrophotometer using the appropriate substrates 6PG, G6P, and NADP. If a normal or equivocal result is obtained the test should be repeated a few weeks later if the clinical suspicion of G6PD deficiency is great. If necessary the nature of any defect can be studied in more detail using electrophoretic techniques.

3.10 Haemoglobin

Haemoglobin (Hb) is made up of:

1 Haem — a porphyrin ring containing ferrous iron.

2 Globin — a protein made up of polypeptide chains of different lengths and amino acid sequences, the most important being designated α, β, γ, δ. In each molecule there are two α-chains and two non-α chains and to each chain a haem moiety is attached.

The most commonly occurring haemoglobins are:

$\alpha_2\beta_2$ = HbA
$\alpha_2\gamma_2$ = HbF
$\alpha_2\delta_2$ = HbA_2

but other normal haemoglobins are found in early embryonic life. The major haemoglobin of fetal life is HbF, but at birth HbA synthesis is well established. HbF production declines rapidly during the first year but persists into adult life at a very low level. HbA_2 is a minor adult haemoglobin.

The function of the complete haemoglobin molecule is to pick up alveolar oxygen, transport it to the tissues, and then release it for use in metabolism. The sigmoid oxygen dissociation curve of the haemoglobin tetramer reflects this function and contrasts with

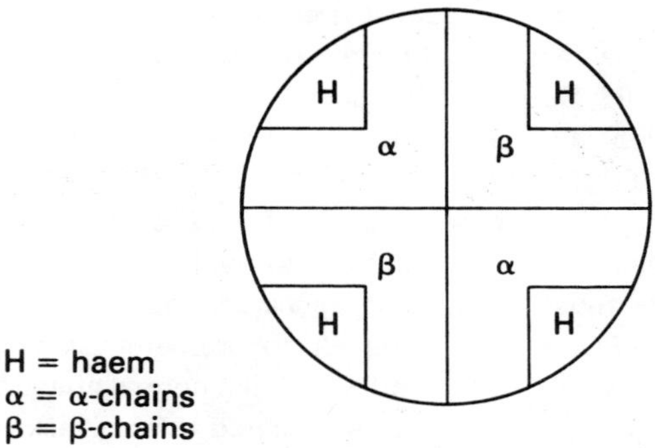

Fig. 3.5 The haemoglobin A molecule.

Table 3.8 Haemoglobin proportions.

	At birth	After two years
HbF	50–90%	<1%
HbA	10–50%	97%
HbA_2	Negligible	1.5–3.0%

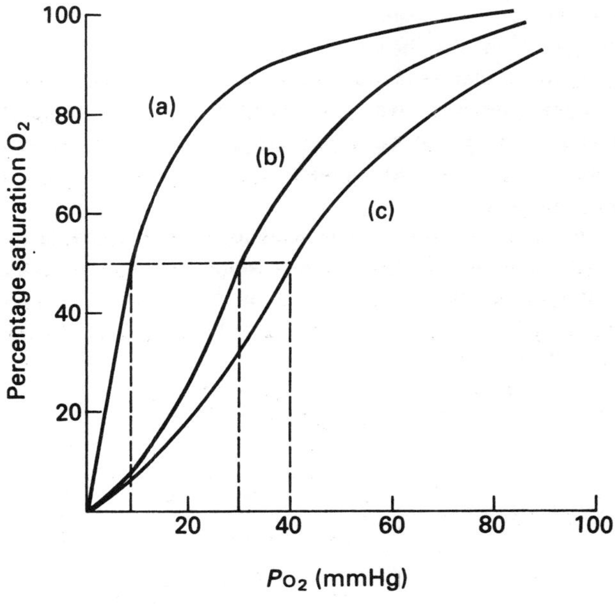

Fig. 3.6 The oxygen dissociation curve.
(a) High affinity (left shift), P_{50} = 10 mmHg.
(b) Normal, P_{50} = 28 mmHg.
(c) Low affinity (right shift), P_{50} = 40 mmHg.

the hyperbolic curve of haemoglobin monomer. Different haemoglobins may have different dissociation curves, and high-affinity haemoglobins are said to show a shift to the left, while those with low affinity show a shift to the right. The oxygen dissociation curve is also affected by the concentration of 2,3-DPG, a high concentration causing a shift to the right, and this glycolytic product helps to modulate the body's response to anaemia. For a given curve the $P\text{O}_2$ giving 50% saturation is known as the P_{50}.

Haemoglobin abnormalities are of two principal types:

1 Failure of normal haemoglobin synthesis giving rise to chain imbalance, which is the hallmark of the thalassaemias. This may be due to many different types of genetic defect.

2 Structural haemoglobin abnormalities, usually due to single point mutations in the gene sequence resulting in new amino acid substitutions within the basic globin chains.

These may affect:

- Haemoglobin solubility (sickle cell disease due to HbSS).
- Oxygen-carrying potential (polycythaemia due to Hb Heathrow).
- Haemoglobin stability (haemolysis due to Hb Köln).

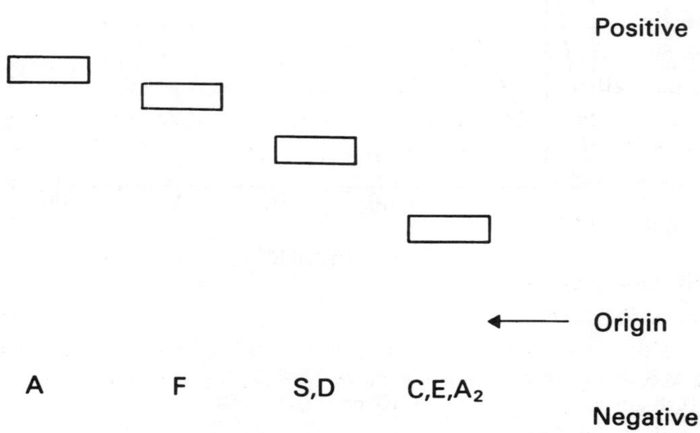

Fig. 3.7 Haemoglobin electrophoresis at pH 8.6 (tris-EDTA borate buffer) on cellulose acetate.

- The ferrous iron in haem (methaemoglobinaemia due to HbM).
- Chain length and synthesis (thalassaemia due to Hb Constant Spring).

or may be of no clinical consequence.

If the mutation affects molecular charge it will also affect electrophoretic mobility.

Haemoglobin electrophoresis

Haemoglobins are charged proteins, and when subjected to electrophoresis at appropriate pH they separate according to their relative charges. For screening purposes electrophoresis of red cell haemolysates on cellulose acetate at pH 8.6 is in general clinical use. Separated haemoglobins may be quantitated by elution and spectrophotometric measurement.

To identify haemoglobins which do not separate by this technique it is necessary to alter the conditions. For instance, using agarose gel at pH 6, S separates from D, C separates from E, and a clearer separation between A and F is obtained. For the last-mentioned distinction the alkaline denaturation test is more convenient.

The sickle test

HbS has reduced solubility in the deoxygenated state and damages the red cell which contains it so that precipitation takes place. A solubility test for HbS is available commercially. It is very specific for HbS but may not be clearly positive when the patient is very anaemic. A positive result should always be followed by Hb electrophoresis to confirm the diagnosis.

HbA_2 quantitation

This can be performed by elution from cellulose acetate electrophoretic strips or by microchromatography using an ion exchange resin (DEAE cellulose). In either case spectrophotometric quantitation of separated HbA_2 is performed.

- HbA_2 is increased in the majority of cases of β-thalassaemia minor.

HbF detection and quantitation

- HbF is resistant to both acid and alkaline denaturation.

Acid elution test for HbF in red cells (Kleihauer)

A peripheral blood film is fixed in ethanol and treated with an acid buffer. HbA elutes from the cells but HbF remains and can be stained with eosin. If HbF is present it is usually randomly distributed throughout the cells so that some are positive and some are negative. In hereditary persistence of HbF (HP HF) however, there is an even distribution of HbF throughout the cells in most cases.

The Kleihauer test is useful in:

- The detection of fetal blood — prevention of rhesus disease, antenatal diagnostic techniques, and forensic work.
- The diagnosis of HP HF and its differential diagnosis (*see below*).

Alkaline denaturation test

If a haemolysate is treated with sodium hydroxide, HbA is denatured and may be precipitated by the addition of ammonium sulphate. The HbA is filtered out and the HbF, which is present in the filtrate, is quantitated spectrophotometrically.

- Normal adult blood contains less than 2% HbF.

Causes of an increase of HbF after two years of age include:

- β-Thalassaemia.
- Sickle cell disease.
- Aplastic anaemia (including Fanconi's anaemia).
- Malignant or premalignant conditions of the myeloid stem cell (including juvenile chronic myeloid leukaemia).
- Paroxysmal nocturnal haemoglobinuria (PNH).
- Hereditary persistence of HbF (HP HF).

Oxygen dissociation curve (*see* p. 71)

This test is usually performed to exclude a haemoglobin variant as a cause of unexplained polycythaemia.

Haemoglobin stability

Unstable haemoglobins can be detected by placing them under some form of stress, such as heat, which normal haemoglobin is better able to withstand. These tests are not very reliable.

Haemoglobin M

Methaemoglobin (met-Hb) may be detected electrophoretically or spectroscopically, and the distinction between met-HbA and met-HbM can be made by treating the met-Hb with various chemicals.

Cyanosis from birth or childhood in the absence of cardiopulmonary disease is good circumstantial evidence of the presence of HbM or $NADH_2$ met-Hb reductase deficiency, and further investigation should be undertaken by specialized laboratories.

Protein chemistry and molecular biology

Modern techniques of globin chain analysis and, more recently, recombinant DNA technology have led to important advances in the understanding and diagnosis of haemoglobin abnormalities. In particular, they have enabled antenatal diagnosis to be offered to families at risk of sickle cell disease and thalassaemia major, some cases being diagnosable in the first trimester of pregnancy using chorionic villus biopsy.

3.11 Blood transfusion and immunohaematology

The purpose of laboratory testing in blood transfusion is to choose suitable donors and protect their health while selecting safe, compatible blood products for the recipients. Potential donors are therefore required to answer simple questions on their general health, and those likely to transmit diseases such as malaria, hepatitis or AIDS may be excluded on these grounds alone. Before blood is taken a rough check of haemoglobin concentration is made, and all acceptable donor units are tested for hepatitis B surface antigen (HBsAg), antibodies to human immunodeficiency virus (HIV) and for evidence of infection with syphilis before they are used. Now that blood is taken into sealed plastic containers infection introduced after venepuncture is very uncommon. Since the red cells are the most important and potentially the most immediately dangerous therapeutic element of the blood, the majority of subsequent work in routine blood transfusion is devoted to their analysis. This is largely achieved by the use of specific antibodies to red cell antigens, which may be naturally occurring, arise as a consequence of disease or medical treatment, or are specially prepared for the purpose. These methods are also used in the diagnosis and management of diseases such as autoimmune haemolytic anaemia (AIHA) and haemolytic disease of the newborn (HDN). As the use of organ and bone marrow transplantation has expanded, so the analysis of white cell and platelet antigens has grown in importance, and these are now extensively studied. Some antigenic systems found in serum proteins are also recognized.

Red cells, antigens and antibodies

The red cell membrane is negatively charged, and this charge keeps the cells separated from each other. In order to cause agglutination, an antibody must be able to bridge the gap between red cells and, when they are in saline suspension, IgM is able to do this while IgG cannot.

Within the membrane are many different chemical antigens capable of stimulating an immune response. The resulting antibodies are usually IgM or IgG, and each type has different properties.

- IgM antibodies act best in the cold at 4 °C, but may act in the warm if they have a wide thermal range. They are 'complete', causing direct agglutination of red cells in saline, and are capable of fixing complement and causing complement-mediated haemolysis. Because of their size they do not cross the placenta. They are often 'naturally occurring'.
- IgG antibodies act best at 37 °C and are 'incomplete' so that no agglutination occurs when they are mixed with red cells in saline. Agglutination can be brought about by reducing the negative

Table 3.9 Blood group antibodies.

	IgM	IgG
Temperature	Cold	Warm
Complement fixation	Yes	Yes or no
Haemolysis	Yes	Rarely haemolytic
Agglutination	Complete	Incomplete
Incidence	Naturally occurring	Immune
Placental transfer	No	Yes
Typical example	Anti-A or B	Anti-D

charges which separate the cells (enzyme treatment, albumin addition, low ionic strength media) or by bridging the gap between the cells with an anti-human globulin (antiglobulin or Coombs' test). IgG antibodies are less efficient at fixing complement than IgM antibodies, but they are capable of crossing the placenta. They do not usually occur 'naturally' and have to be induced by immune stimulation. They are therefore often described as 'immune antibodies'.

The ABO system

The ABO antigens are glycosphingolipids which are present, but not fully developed, at birth. Antigen specificity is due to the terminal carbohydrate portion of the molecule, and inheritance is autosomal, A and B being dominant and O being amorphic.

Antibodies within the ABO system are usually IgM 'naturally occurring' and complete, but are not present at birth and probably develop in response to infection with bacteria which share similar antigenic structures. Antibodies only develop to the antigens which the subject lacks. Some individuals develop 'immune' antibodies, especially when stimulated by incompatible transfusion or pregnancy, and such antibodies may be IgM or IgG.

The ABO antigens are present on the surface of red cells, white cells and platelets, and are also found in the body fluids of the 80% of the population who are 'secretors'.

3.11 Blood transfusion and immunohaematology

Table 3.10 The ABO system.

Genotype	Phenotype	Antibodies	Percentage in U.K.
OO	O	Anti-A (α) Anti-B (β)	47
AO AA	A	Anti-B (β)	40
BO BB	B	Anti-A (α)	10
AB	AB	—	3

A number of variants are recognized within the ABO system, especially within A. Thus A_1, A_2, A_3, A_m, etc. are described, depending on the cell reactions with various antisera.

The rhesus (Rh) system

Rhesus antigens are membrane proteins, the most important of which is designated D. The 85% of the population possessing this antigen are known as 'rhesus-positive' and the other 15% as 'rhesus-negative'. Among the other antigens in the Rh complex the most important are the alleles C, c, and E, e, but d is amorphic. D itself has a complex structure, so that D variants occur and weak forms of D are also recognized (Du). The principal rhesus complexes and their shorthand notations are shown below.

Antigen complex	*Notation*
CDe	R1
cDE	R2
cDe	Ro
CDE	RZ
cde	r
Cde	r′
cdE	r″
CdE	ry

The commonest complexes are R1, R2, and r. Notations with capital R are rhesus-positive. Notations with a small r are rhesus-negative.

Rhesus antibodies are *not* 'naturally occurring' but are 'immune' IgG antibodies formed in response to transfusion with incompatible blood or by placental transfer of incompatible fetal red cells. They are typical incomplete antibodies and are able to cross the placenta, anti-D being the commonest cause of haemolytic disease of the newborn (HDN). Other Rh antibodies may also cause HDN, and warm autoimmune haemolytic anaemia (AIHA) is often due to antibodies with Rh specificity, especially anti-e.

Some other blood group systems

Lewis (Le). This is a body fluid system, but the antigens are absorbed onto the red cell surface. There is a complex interrelation between H (the substrate for the ABO system) and Se (the secretor gene). Antibodies are naturally occurring and are usually IgM and bind complement, but transfusion reactions are rare.

P. One of the important features of this complex system is that the IgG Donath–Landsteiner antibody found in paroxysmal cold haemoglobinuria (PCH) has P specificity.

Ii. Neonatal cord blood samples show i specificity, but this declines and is largely replaced by I at 18 months of age. Autoimmune haemolytic anaemia due to anti-I occurs in cold agglutinin disease and mycoplasma pneumonia, the antibody being IgM. Anti-i is sometimes found in infectious mononucleosis.

Kell. These antigens are important because they give rise to IgG antibodies which may cause HDN and haemolytic transfusion reactions. There is an association between rare Kell groups and chronic granulomatous disease.

Duffy. This system is also associated with HDN and haemolytic transfusion reactions. Antibodies may be difficult to detect save by the antiglobulin technique. Duffy-negative red cells appear to be immune to *Plasmodium vivax* infection, and this genotype is common in West Africa.

Kidd antibodies may also be difficult to demonstrate. They fix complement and may cause serious transfusion reactions, which are sometimes delayed.

Serology techniques

Samples for blood group serology are taken into plain sterile glass tubes and allowed to clot at room temperature. Where AIHA due to cold antibodies is suspected, samples should be maintained at 37 °C from collection until separation is complete. Blood for direct antiglobulin testing may be taken into EDTA (Sequestrene).

Complete antibodies

Cells in saline suspension and serum are mixed together at 20 °C and left undisturbed for one or two hours.

Incomplete antibodies

Agglutination can be induced by:

- Enzyme addition.
- Albumin addition.
- Antiglobulin technique (indirect).
- Antiglobulin technique (direct).

Further identification of the type of antibody or complement attached to the red cells can be achieved by using AHG specific for IgG types and complement components.

Blood grouping

ABO. Patient or donor cells are mixed with specific anti-A, anti-B and high-titre O antisera. Specific known A, B, and O cells are mixed with patient or donor serum.

Rhesus. Patient or donor cells are mixed with one or more specific anti-D antisera.

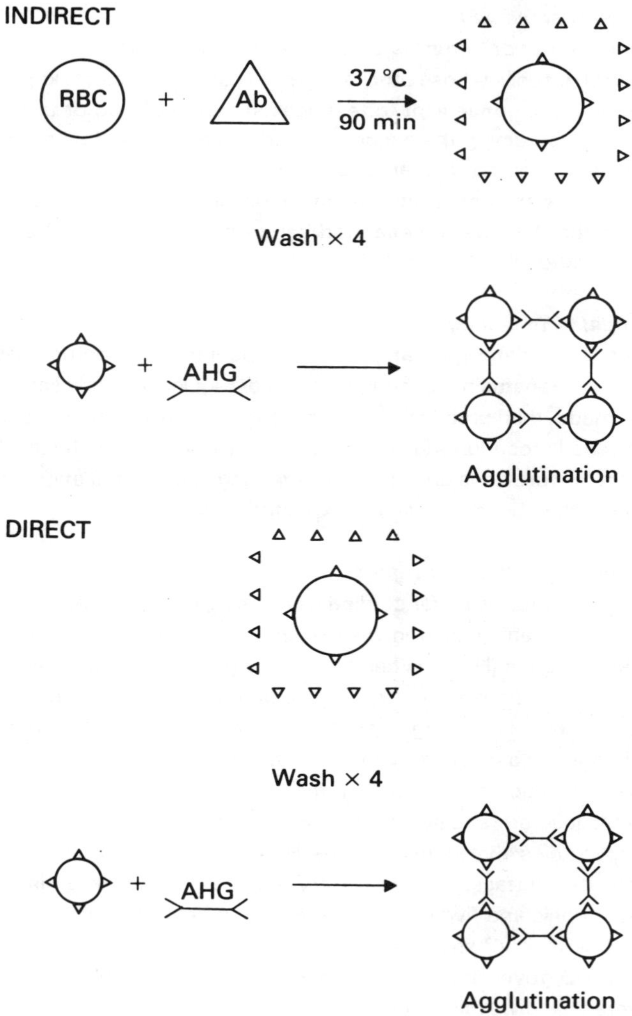

Fig. 3.8 The antiglobulin technique.

Antibody screening
Patient or donor serum is studied by testing it against a panel of group O red cells whose other antigenic characteristics are known. It is often more convenient to test against a pool of two or three cell samples containing the majority of red cell antigens. If an autoantibody is suspected then an eluate can be made from the sensitized cells to assist in antibody identification. If a cold autoantibody is suspected then warm separated serum should be titrated against pooled group O red cells.

Compatibility testing
It is still mandatory to carry out a compatibility test before issuing blood for transfusion, although the use of regular antibody screening has made this practice less vital and has assisted the use of shortened procedures in an emergency. The purpose of the test is to detect any previous error in sample testing and identification and to confirm the absence of any unexpected incompatibility.

Histocompatibility antigens
All animal species so far studied have a single major transplantation antigen system, which in man is known as the human lymphatic antigen system (HLA). When tissue or organ grafting is undertaken, graft survival depends on the degree of match of the HLA system. It is also clear that a large variety of chronic diseases of uncertain aetiology are associated with a particular HLA.

The genetic loci governing the development of HLA antigen specificities are situated on the short arm of chromosome 6. The glycoproteins that constitute the HLA antigens are present on all tissue cell surfaces except for erythrocytes. The system is highly polymorphic and five major gene loci have been described:

- HLA-A, -B, -C antigens are present in most tissues.
- HLA-D governs the proliferative response of lymphocytes from different individuals when mixed together (mixed lymphocyte culture, MLC).
- HLA-DR is detected only on B-lymphocytes and monocytes and

is very closely related to the D locus.

- HLA-D and -DR are often equated with the immune response genes of animals and are often called Ia antigens.
- HLA-A, -B, -C and -DR are detected by complement–dependent microlymphocytotoxicity.
- HLA-D is detected by the MLC reaction.

Any individual inherits from each parent the corresponding HLA chromosomal region with its particular gene (allele) at each locus, the combined genetic information constituting the HLA haplotype. There are a large number of different determinants which between them can generate more than 30 million distinguishable combinations.

The distribution of allele frequencies is relatively even, with few frequencies over 10% but many of up to 5%. These frequencies are such that in any typical Caucasian population 75% of individuals will have four different HLA-A and -B antigens. Because of the close linkage between loci, however, within families 25% of siblings will be HLA identical.

This has important implications if an HLA-typed panel is being set up for bone marrow donation or to prepare matched platelets for transfusion.

Table 3.11 HLA and disease.

Disease	Antigen	Frequency (%) in patients	Frequency (%) in controls
Acute lymphocytic leukaemia	A2	63	37
Hodgkin's disease	BW 35	25	16
Hodgkin's disease	A1	39	32
Hodgkin's disease	B8	26	22
Pernicious anaemia	B7	43	25
Haemochromatosis	A3	72	21

HLA and disease

Possible mechanisms of association include:

- Immune response genes closely associated with the HLA system.
- Molecular mimicry. This hypothesis assumes that HLA antigens resemble the antigenic structure of specific infectious agents, inducing cross-tolerance.
- HLA antigens may act as receptor sites for viral or hormone attachment.

HLA and bone marrow transplants

As with organ transplantation, the results of transplantation of bone marrow from an identical twin (syngeneic) in leukaemia and aplastic anaemia are very good with virtually no graft versus host reaction.

Allogeneic transplantation using a sibling donor – recipient combination with an identical HLA match and MLC non-reactivity is still complicated by a significant incidence of GVHD. This indicates that other, as yet unidentified, histocompatibility systems must be important.

Granulocytes

These cells persist longer in the circulation of the recipient if there is HLA and ABO compatibility between donor and recipient. However, provided there are no leucocyte antibodies present, there is no evidence that incompatibility impairs function.

Platelets

HLA-compatible platelets show a significantly increased *in vivo* survival, but it is uncertain whether length of survival equates with efficacy. The only true test of function is the clinical effect. In general, leukaemic patients receiving cytotoxics are immunosuppressed and do not form antibodies readily. Random donor platelets are satisfactory in the majority of instances. The refractory patient with thrombocytopenia can, however, be supported long-term with

HLA-matched platelets from related and non-related donors by harvesting from these donors using one of the cell separators.

In addition to ABO and HLA antigens platelets bear specific antigens such as those of the PLA system. Alloantibodies may develop and cause fetal thrombocytopenia by a mechanism analogous to that of HDN and are also capable of causing severe thrombocytopenia in affected subjects following blood transfusion (post-transfusion purpura).

Serum groups

Antibodies to serum groups such as the immunoglobulin Gm group sometimes cause minor transfusion reactions.

3.12 Haemostasis

The haemostatic mechanism protects the body from excessive blood loss after injury but has to be controlled to prevent the propagation of thrombus, which might occlude the blood supply to vital structures. The process continues from the moment of endothelial damage until the completion of repair.

The main components of the mechanism are:

1 The vessel walls.

2 The platelets.

3 Fibrin formation (coagulation).

4 Fibrinolysis.

Although considered separately, these four aspects of haemostasis are all activated at the moment of injury, and they work in a coordinated and interrelated way to achieve their objective.

The vessel wall

Vessels may contract reflexly or in response to humoral stimuli. The subendothelial surface is responsible for haemostatic activation, and endothelial cell products include:

- Prostacyclin (PGI_2), which affects platelet function.
- Part of the factor VIII molecule complex (VWF) necessary for platelet adhesion.

- Fibrinolytic activator.

There are no commonly used simple tests of vessel wall function, though its contribution to platelet function, coagulation, and fibrinolysis can be measured. Examples of disorders affecting the vessel wall are:

- Hereditary telangiectasia.
- Ehlers–Danlos syndrome.
- Scurvy.
- Von Willebrand's disease.

The platelets

The morphological appearance of platelets under the light microscope has already been considered on p. 53. Under the electron microscope the following important features may be noted:

1 The platelet membrane, which contains:

- Platelet factor 3 (PF3), a phospholipid of importance in coagulation (instrinsic system).

2 Dense bodies, whose contents include:

- ADP, ATP, serotonin and calcium.

3 α-Granules, whose contents include:

- Platelet factor 4 (PF4) (heparin neutralizing factor).
- β-Thromboglobulin (β-TG) (a platelet-specific protein structurally related to PF4).
- VWF.
- Fibrinogen and fibronectin.

4 Actomyosin fibres beneath the cell membrane which are responsible for clot retraction.

When platelets are activated they:

1 Change their shape from discs to spiny spheres.

2 Adhere to subendothelial collagen in the presence of VWF.

3 Aggregate by adhering to each other.

4 Release the contents of their granules, thus stimulating further adhesion and aggregation.

5 Take part in clot retraction.

The metabolic pathways by which platelets undergo these changes and interact with the vessel wall involve the metabolism of phospholipid via arachidonic acid to prostaglandins and thromboxanes. In the

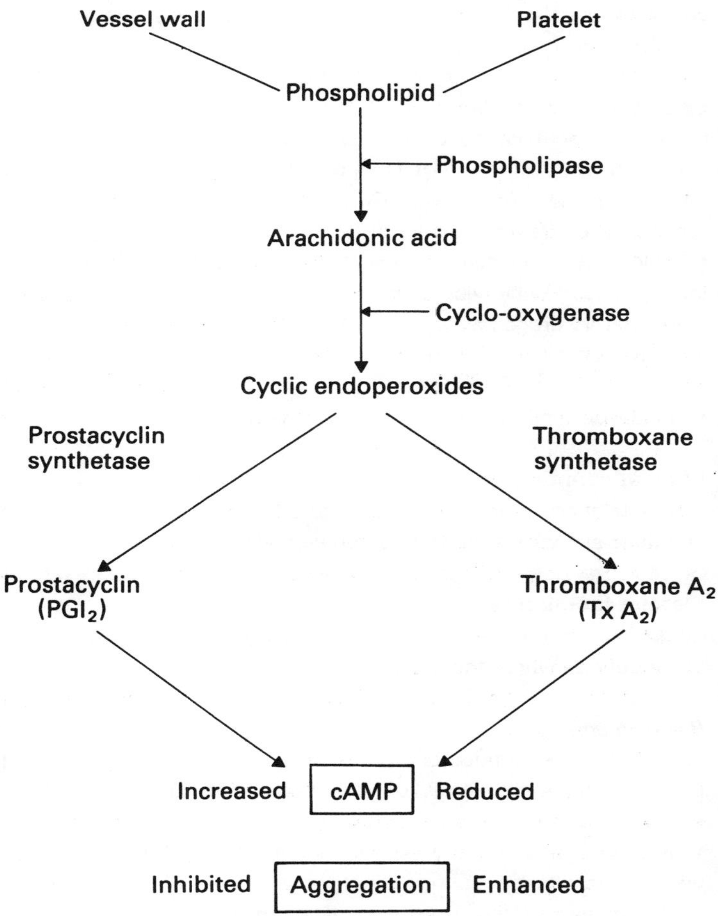

Fig. 3.9 Platelet–vessel wall interaction.

vessel wall prostacyclin (PGI_2) is produced, and this inhibits platelet aggregation, whereas in the platelet thromboxane A_2 (TxA_2) is produced, and this promotes platelet aggregation. These properties are mediated by their effect on cyclic AMP (cAMP) and calcium ions within the platelet. The principal steps in the pathways are shown in Fig. 3.9.

Inhibitors of platelet function

- Aspirin (acetylsalicylic acid) acetylates cyclo-oxygenase and causes irreversible failure of TxA_2 synthesis for the life-span of the affected platelet. Vessel wall PGI_2 synthesis is also affected but can recover when treatment is stopped.
- Sulphinpyrazone causes reversible inhibition of cyclo-oxygenase. Indomethacin, phenylbutazone and other non-steroidal anti-inflammatory drugs have a similar effect.
- Dipyridamole is a phosphodiesterase inhibitor and increases cAMP.
- Imidazole inhibits thromboxane synthetase.

Platelet counting

The platelet count and the causes and effects of thrombocytopenia and thrombocytosis are considered elsewhere.

Platelet function tests

Routine tests of platelet function are designed to analyse haemostatic defects where the platelet count is fairly normal.

Bleeding time

This is a rather crude, but very useful, *in vivo* test of platelet function. The normal range is 2–9 minutes. The patient should:

- Not have severe thrombocytopenia.
- Not have ingested any aspirin-containing drug for at least two weeks before testing.
- Be warned of the possibility of a small scar remaining after healing.

An abnormal result is obtained in von Willebrand's disease and in most qualitative platelet disorders.

- The bleeding time is not a test of coagulation and is normal in haemophilia.

Platelet aggregation

Various agonists are added at appropriate concentrations to platelet-rich plasma (PRP), and as the platelets aggregrate the optical density decreases.

The primary phase of aggregation is due to the effect of the aggregating agent itself, but the secondary phase is due to the release reaction of the treated platelets and is therefore irreversible. The most commonly used agonists are ADP, adrenaline, arachidonic acid, collagen and ristocetin. Collagen and ristocetin do not show a primary phase.

Spontaneous aggregation of stirred PRP takes place in some myeloproliferative disorders, especially when the platelet count is elevated.

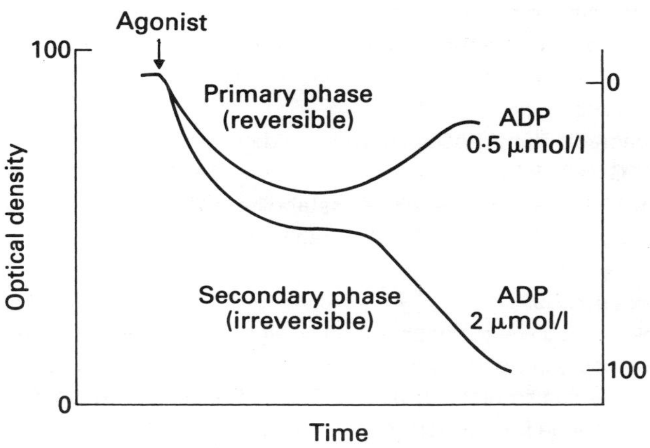

Fig. 3.10 Platelet aggregation traces.

Table 3.12 Platelet aggregation findings.

	Agonist		
Condition	ADP	Collagen	Ristocetin
Aspirin or aspirin-like defect	P	R	N
Storage pool disease	P	R	N
Glanzmann's thrombasthenia	A	A	N
Bernard–Soulier syndrome	N	N	R or A
von Willebrand's disease	N	N	N, R, or A

N = normal; P = primary phase only; R = reduced; A = absent.

Platelet antibodies

Immunofluorescent and enzyme-linked immunoassay (ELISA) techniques have improved the detection of platelet antibodies in the diagnosis of thrombocytopenia.

Platelet ADP and ATP

Firefly extract is luminous in the presence of ATP, and assays have been devised to measure platelet total nucleotides and release. This is of value in the diagnosis of storage pool disease.

Platelet products

Immunoradiometric assays have been devised for:

- β-TG and PF4.
- Thromboxane B_2 (the stable metabolite of TxA_2).
- Prostaglandin 6-keto-$F_{1\alpha}$ (the stable metabolite of PGI_2).

Platelet survival

Platelets circulate for approximately eight days under normal circumstances, but platelet life-span is markedly reduced in thrombocytopenia due to platelet destruction or pooling (*see* p. 257). The best technique for measurement of platelet survival involves the use of the radioactive isotope indium-111 to label platelets which are then reinjected.

3.12 Haemostasis

Coagulation

When blood clots, fibrin is laid down within and around the primary haemostatic plug created by platelet adhesion and aggregation. Fibrin is formed from circulating inert fibrinogen by the action of thrombin and as a result of a complex series of enzymatic reactions which begin with tissue damage and the exposure of subendothelial collagen. As each clotting factor is activated to a serine protease, it attacks its substrate, and an amplified chain reaction takes place, culminating in the explosive generation of thrombin at the site of injury. At the same time a number of modulating positive and negative feedback reactions take place and various circulating inhibitory proteins ensure that the process does not spread too far.

In the laboratory there are two basic methods of activating coagulation, known as the intrinsic and extrinsic systems. *In vivo* they act together and are probably more interrelated than the original laboratory tests suggested.

The intrinsic system

When placed in a glass tube, blood clots in about 10 minutes due to the surface contact activity of the glass itself. This is probably analogous to exposure of subendothelial collagen *in vivo*. The contact factors then interact in a complex way, and factor XIa stimulates factor IX which, in the presence of factor VIII, activates factor X. The final common pathway to fibrin production through factors V and II (prothrombin) then completes the process.

The extrinsic system

When a tissue such as brain is added to citrated plasma the plasma clots rapidly after recalcification, a phenomenon which is probably related *in vivo* to tissue damage. The tissue factor activates factor VII, which then activates factor X, leading into the final common pathway. It was soon realized that the intrinsic pathway is the more important clinically, since the severe coagulation disorders due to factor VIII and IX deficiency (haemophilias A and B) show no abnormality of the extrinsic system.

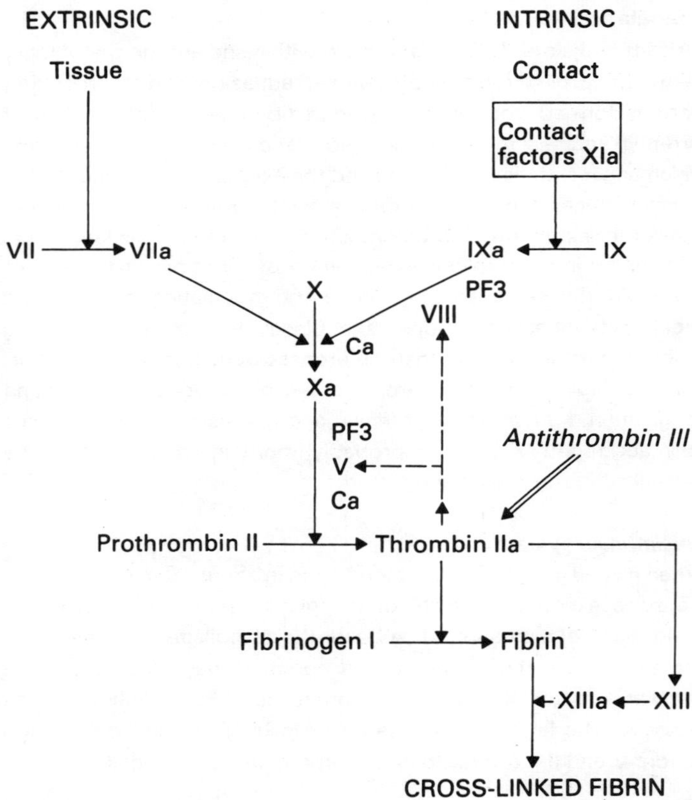

Fig. 3.11 The coagulation mechanism.

The contact factors

Factor XII is activated by contact and stimulates factor XI in the presence of prekallikrein (Fletcher factor) and high molecular weight kininogen (Fitzgerald factor). Factor XIa activates factor IX.

Factor VIII

The molecular weight of factor VIII is greater than 10^6, and it is composed of an X-linked and an autosomal part. The X-linked part is known as VIII:C because it contains the clotting activity which is missing in haemophilia A and is lost during the clotting of normal blood. Its stable antigenic counterpart is known as VIII:CAg. The site of synthesis is unknown but includes the liver. The autosomal part is known as von Willebrand factor (VWF) because it is lacking in von Willebrand's disease. It is a multimeric protein, the higher molecular weight multimers being responsible for ristocetin-induced platelet aggregation. VWF is synthesized in endothelium and megakaryocytes, and is therefore found in platelets, where it plays an important part in platelet–vessel wall interaction. VWF also has a role in the stabilization of VIII:C in the circulation.

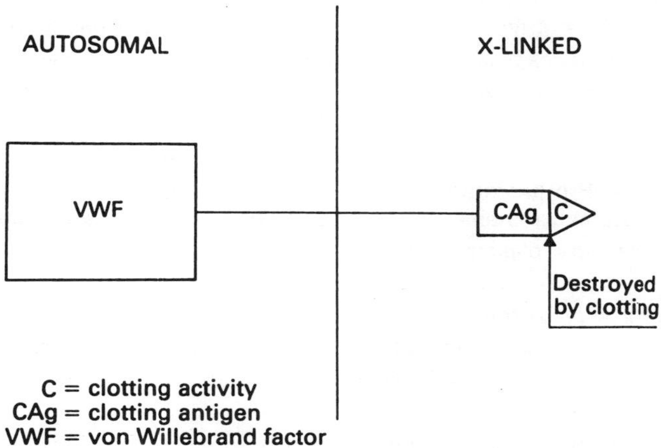

Fig. 3.12 The factor VIII molecule.

The vitamin K-dependent factors

Factors II, VII, IX, X and proteins C and S depend on vitamin K for the completion of their synthesis. The step involved is the γ-carboxylation of glutamic acid residues, a modification which is essential for calcium binding. The reaction is inhibited by oral anticoagulants such as warfarin. Protein C, when activated, inhibits the activity of factors V and VIII:C, a reaction for which protein S is a cofactor.

Thrombin

Thrombin is a powerful serine protease which converts fibrinogen to fibrin. It stimulates factors V and VIII before eventually denaturing and inhibiting them. It is also the activator of factor XIII (*see* Fig. 3.11).

Antithrombin III is the most important serine protease inhibitor and is particularly active against thrombin and factor Xa. The speed of its reaction is markedly enhanced by heparin.

Fibrinogen

Fibrinogen is a dimer, each monomer consisting of three polypeptide chains, α, β and γ. The thrombin cleavage site is at the Aα and Bβ portions of the α- and β-chains, and following the loss of the A- and B-peptides the fibrin polymerizes. Fibrin stabilization is achieved by the transamidase factor XIIIa, especially through cross-linking of the γ-chains.

Coagulation tests

The starting material for all routine coagulation tests is citrated platelet-poor plasma (PPP).

Prothrombin test (PT)

- The extrinsic system is tested. A clot forms in about 13 seconds in normal subjects and the result is expressed as a ratio of the normal control.

Test sample = 26 seconds
Control sample = 13 seconds
PT ratio (PTR) = 2.0

Thromboplastins are standardized by an internationally recognized system. The test is sensitive to deficiencies of factors VII, X, V, II, I.

Important causes of an abnormal PTR are:

- Vitamin K deficiency.
- Oral anticoagulation.
- Liver disease.
- Congenital deficiency of sensitive factors.

- Diffuse intravascular coagulation (DIC).

The PT is not very sensitive to heparin.

- The PT is *normal* in haemophilia A (factor VIII deficiency) and haemophilia B (factor IX deficiency — Christmas disease) and in contact factor deficiencies.
- The coagulation inhibitor associated with SLE is most conveniently detected by performing the PT using brain extract diluted 1/250 or 1/500. The clotting time is substantially prolonged compared to a control sample. Other tests using kaolin (intrinsic system) and Russell's viper venom (factor X activator) are also used.

Thrombotest

This commercial test was developed primarily for the control of oral anticoagulant therapy.

Kaolin cephalin clotting test (KCCT)/kaolin partial thromboplastin test (KPTT)/activated PTT (APTT)

- The intrinsic system is tested.

A clot forms in about 40 seconds.

The test is sensitive to deficiencies of factors XII, Fletcher, Fitzgerald, XI, IX, VIII, X, V, II, I. Important causes of a prolonged KCCT/KPPT are:

- Congenital deficiency of sensitive factors (especially haemophilia).
- Lupus anticoagulant.
- Heparin therapy.
- Liver disease.
- DIC.

The KCCT/KPTT is:

- Not very sensitive to vitamin K deficiency and oral anticoagulation.
- Normal in factor VII deficiency.
- Sometimes shortened in early or compensated DIC and in some prothrombotic states.

The thrombin test (TT)

• The final reaction in which fibrinogen is converted to fibrin is tested.

A clot forms in about 10 seconds. The test is sensitive to fibrinogen abnormalities, the presence of fibrinogen degradation products (FDPs), and to the presence of heparin.

Important causes of a prolonged TT are:

- Hypofibrinogenaemia.
- Dysfibrinogenaemia.
- Heparin therapy.
- DIC.

Reptilase test

This snake venom converts fibrinogen to a form of fibrin independently of thrombin. The presence of heparin does not affect its activity significantly. The reptilase time is prolonged in the same circumstances as the thrombin time except that heparinized plasma gives a normal result.

Identification of factor deficiencies

A combination of clinical information and screening test results will often allow a provisional diagnosis to be made. Further investigation depends on the resources available, but mixing experiments with known deficient plasmas are very useful in the identification of the

Table 3.13 Coagulation screening test abnormalities.

Condition	PT	KCCT	TT	Reptilase
Vitamin K deficiency, oral anticoagulants	A	a	N	N
Haemophilia	N	a or A	N	N
Liver disease	a or A	a or A	N or a	N or a
Heparin	a	A	A	N
DIC	a or A	a or A	a or A	a or A

N = normal; A = abnormal; a = mildly abnormal.

deficient factor(s). Inhibitors can also be detected by mixing experiments using normal plasma.

Factor assays

Most clotting factors are assayed by their ability to correct the clotting times of known deficient plasmas. Specific factor assays should always be used to confirm a congenital haemostatic defect suspected because of the clinical findings and/or screening tests.

- Occasionally the screening tests are normal despite the presence of a significant defect. Careful judgement is needed before deciding how to pursue a doubtful case.

Factor VIII:C assay

Two methods are available:

1 The one-stage method is a KCCT-based assay using totally deficient plasma from a patient with severe haemophilia A or a similar artificially prepared plasma.

2 The two-stage method begins with the production of factor Xa from a plasma dilution in the presence of serum, factor V and PF3. In the second stage the Xa is used to produce a clot, the clotting time being dependent on the concentration of factor VIII:C in the original plasma.

Factor VIII:CAg assay

The antigenic part of the factor VIII:C molecule is recognized by the non-precipitating antibodies which develop in treated haemophiliacs. Most haemophiliacs also lack factor VIII:CAg, but unlike factor VIII:C it is present in serum. The test's principal value is in antenatal diagnosis.

VWF: Ag assay

Antibodies to VWF are raised in rabbits or other species and VWF: Ag is usually measured by immunoelectrophoresis. These antibodies can also be used to study VWF: Ag after it has first been electrophoresed through a non-antibody-containing agarose gel to produce multimer separation on the basis of molecular size.

Table 3.14 Factor VIII values. The normal range for all types of factor VIII is approximately 50–200% of pooled normal control.

	C	CAg	VWF:Ag	VWF
Normal plasma	N	N	N	N
Normal serum	A	N or R	N	N
Haemophilia A	R or A	R or A	N	N
von Willebrand's disease	R	R	R	R

N = normal; R = reduced; A = absent.
VIII:CAg is often rather lower in normal serum than normal plasma.
VIII:CAg is occasionally normal or near normal in haemophilia A.
Von Willebrand's disease shows great variability in all its findings.
All VIII values tend to rise in response to inflammation or injury.

VWF assay

Platelets are washed free of VWF and may be preserved by formalin treatment. Dilutions of test and control plasma are added to washed platelets in an aggregometer, and ristocetin is added to the stirred mixture. The slope or OD_{max} of the traces is measured and the value of VWF calculated.

Fibrinogen assay

Various chemical, immunological and clotting methods are available. The normal range is 2.0–4.0 g/l. Fibrinogen concentration is increased in response to inflammation or injury and is reduced in severe DIC and in congenital hypofibrinogenaemia. Where there is acquired or congenital dysfibrinogenaemia the total fibrinogen concentration may be normal despite a prolonged thrombin time.

Antithrombin III

Antithrombin III is measured by chromogenic substrate assays or immunoelectrophoresis. Antithrombin III deficiency is a hereditary condition associated with a thrombotic tendency, and levels below 80% of normal may be clinically significant. Reduced levels are also found in DIC and nephrotic syndrome.

Factor XIII

Factor XIII deficiency is very rare but should be considered in any unexplained haemostatic defect. Clots derived from patients with factor XIII deficiency are unstable in 5 M urea.

Fibrinolysis

Following injury, circulating plasminogen is activated by fibrinolytic activator to the active serine protease plasmin. This enzyme is able to destroy many proteins including fibrinogen, fibrin, factor V and factor VIII. Plasmin is neutralized by a number of inhibitory proteins, the most important of which is α_2-antiplasmin, and this prevents the widespread activation of the fibrinolytic mechanism.

Fibrinolytic activator is present in many tissues and body fluids and is synthesized by endothelium. Urinary activator, or urokinase, can be recovered from the urine, and streptococci manufacture a proactivator, streptokinase, which can form a complex with plasminogen to cause fibrinolytic activation.

Plasmin digests fibrin or fibrinogen to form fibrin (ogen) degradation products (FDPs), which are usually removed from the circulation immediately. If they are produced in excess they may persist in the circulation and are capable of interfering with thrombin-induced fibrinogen to fibrin conversion. The amino acids ε-aminocaproic acid and tranexamic acid inhibit plasminogen activation.

Tests for fibrinolysis

Unless fibrinolytic activation is extreme, antiplasmin is sufficiently powerful to absorb any plasmin released into the circulation. This antiplasmin can be removed by the addition of acetic acid, which precipitates fibrinogen, plasminogen, plasminogen activator, and any free plasmin. The process is called euglobulin precipitation and antiplasmin is left in solution.

Euglobulin clot lysis time

Euglobulin precipitate is clotted with thrombin and the clot maintained at 37 °C and observed. Normally the clot will remain for at least two hours before dissolving, but in the presence of excessive fibrinolysis it may have disappeared within 15 minutes.

Fibrin plate test

A fibrin plate is prepared in a Petri dish and euglobulin precipitates are then dropped onto the surface of the fibrin and incubated overnight. Zones of lysis appear whose diameter gives a semi-quantitiative assessment of plasminogen activator and any free plasmin in the precipitate. If it is desired to measure free plasmin alone, heated plates can be used as they do not contain plasminogen.

Tissue plasminogen activator (tPA) and its inhibitor (PAI)

Chromogenic substrate assays of these more sophisticated tests are now available.

Fibrin(ogen) degradation products (FDPs)

FDPs are conveniently measured by immunological techniques in which antibodies to fibrin(ogen) are linked to latex particles. The sample tube is evacuated and contains thrombin and a fibrinolytic inhibitor which ensure complete clotting of the sample without subsequent lysis of the clot. The serum is tested with antibody-linked latex particles, which flocculate in the presence of FDPs.

FDPs should be less than 10 mg/l in normal plasma and are typically increased in DIC.

Antiplasmin

α_2-Antiplasmin may be measured by chromogenic substrate assay. A deficiency of α_2-antiplasmin is associated with a haemorrhagic tendency.

3.13 Tissue diagnostic procedures

The bone marrow

The bone marrow is the source of the red cells, granulocytes,

Table 3.15 Routine haemostatic screening scheme.

History	Present — nature of bleeding Past — dental — operative Drugs — aspirin
Examination	Joints, muscles, liver, spleen
Haemoglobin and film Platelet count	Bleeding time ? Platelet function tests
PTR KCCT TT	Reptilase ? Correction studies + Factor assays +XIII screen
FDPs ? Euglobulin clot lysis test	

monocytes, platelets and some lymphocytes. In the early stages of development both cell division and differentiation take place, but the capacity to divide is eventually lost and, after further maturation, the completed cells are released into the circulation.

Bone marrow biopsy

Bone marrow can be aspirated by suction or can be removed intact with its bony trabeculae by trephine biopsy. In the adult accessible sites are the manubrium and body of the sternum, the posterior and anterior superior iliac spines and the iliac crest, but trephine samples cannot be taken from the sternum. In children under two years of age the medial aspect of the upper end of the tibia just beneath the tibial tubercle may be used, but in older children biopsies should be taken from the posterior spine or crest.

The procedure is quite safe in experienced hands, but excessive bleeding may take place from the biopsy site in patients with profound thrombocytopenia or severe coagulopathy. Infection of the biopsy site is rare. Bone marrow aspiration alone may be sufficient for the investigation of simple haematinic deficiency and

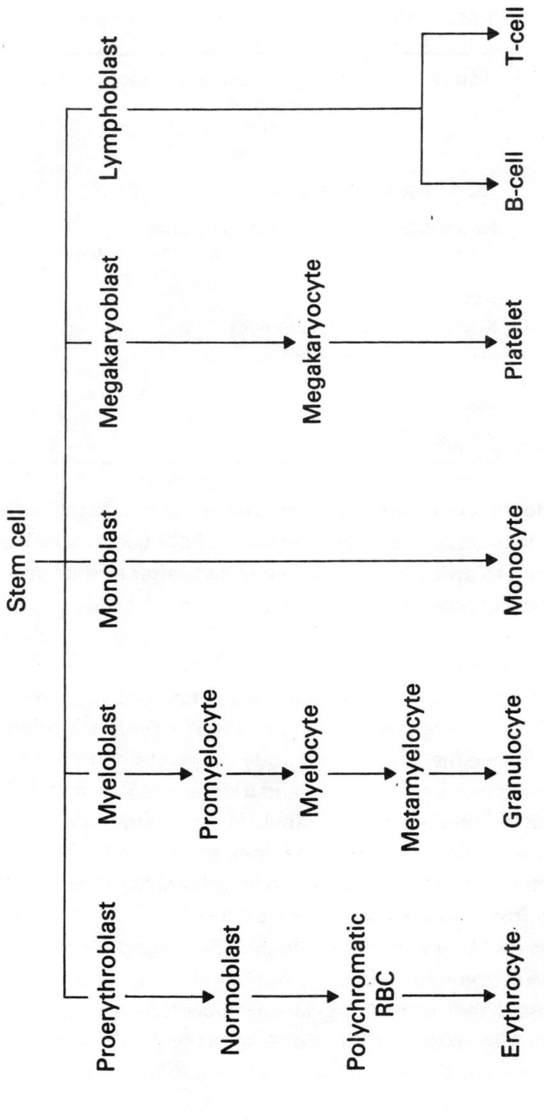

Fig. 3.13 Bone marrow maturation.

obvious cases of leukaemia and myeloma, but many departments now perform trephines routinely in nearly all cases.

Trephine biopsy is especially important for the diagnosis of:

- Myelofibrosis.
- Neoplastic infiltration.
- Lymphoma.
- Aplasia.
- Patients in whom the diagnosis is doubtful.

Processing

Bone marrow aspirates are routinely studied by staining with a Romanowsky dye and with Perl's Prussian blue method for iron.

Special stains are valuable in the differential diagnosis of leukaemia:

- Sudan black or peroxidase is positive in acute myeloid leukaemia because it stains primary azurophilic granules in myeloblasts.
- Periodic acid–Schiff (PAS) shows 'block' positivity in many cases of acute lymphoblastic leukaemia but may give a finer positive reaction in myeloblastic leukaemia. Erythroblasts may be positive in erythroleukaemia.
- A variety of esterase stains are available, and these may be used to differentiate between myeloid, lymphoid, and monocytic leukaemias.

Chloracetate esterase	Myeloid leukaemia
Butyrate esterase	Lymphoid and monocytic leukaemia
Non-specific esterase with fluoride	Monocytic leukaemia
without fluoride	Myeloid leukaemia

- Acid phosphatase is positive in most myeloid and monocytic leukaemia but does differentiate T-cell acute lymphoblastic leukaemia (positive reaction) from other lymphoblastic leukaemia (negative reaction).
- Bone marrow trephines are most satisfactory when embedded in plastic and stained with haematoxylin and eosin. Immunological

analysis of bone marrow trephine samples using immunoperoxidase techniques is helpful when paraffin-embedded sections are analysed.

Examination

The marrow aspirate should be examined under the low and high powers of the microscope. There should normally be:

- Less than 5% blast cells to confirm remission in acute leukaemia.
- Less than 5% plasma cells when excluding a diagnosis of myeloma.
- Less than 20% lymphocytes when excluding a diagnosis of lymphoma.

The morphology of the individual cells must always be considered at the same time.

Myeloma and lymphoma are often very 'patchy' in distribution, and lymphoid follicles occur in normal marrow. Trephine biopsy is invaluable where there is doubt.

The iron stain is studied under the low power to assess the presence or absence of iron in the marrow fragments. The high power is used to look for evidence of increased siderotic granules in maturing normoblasts or for ring sideroblasts, as found in sideroblastic anaemia.

Trephines should be examined carefully under the low power for overall architecture and the relationship of megakaryocytes and any lymphoid follicles to the bony trabeculae. Higher powers are used for fine morphological detail, but the oil immersion lens is rarely required. The reticulin stain is studied for evidence of increased reticulin, which is found in many bone marrow disorders, including myelofibrosis.

Cytogenetics

There are 46 pairs of chromosomes: 44 autosomes and two sex chromosomes — XX, female; XY, male. The chromosomes are

Table 3.16 Important bone marrow findings in non-malignant conditions.

	Iron deficiency	Megaloblastic	Chronic disease	Sideroblastic	Haemolysis	Aplasia
Cellularity	++	+++	+	++	+++	−
Morphology	Hypochromic Microcytic	Megaloblasts Giant metamyelocytes Hypersegmented neutrophils	Defective haemoglobinization	Variable	Macronormoblastic Special features	Empty ± lymphoid increase
Iron	Absent	Increased but no rings	Normal in fragments Reduced in erythrocytes	Ring sideroblasts	May be increased, but usually no rings	

Cellularity key: −, reduced; +, normal; ++, increased; +++, much increased.

Table 3.17 Important bone marrow findings in haematological malignancy.

	ALL	AML	CML	CLL	Lymphoma	Myeloma	Myelofibrosis
Cellularity	+++	+++	+++	++	Variable	Variable	Variable Aspiration difficult
Morphology	Lymphoblasts	Myeloblasts Auer rods	All myeloid series	Lymphocytes	Lymphocytes or lymphoblasts	Plasma cells	Fibrosis ± All myeloid series Megakaryocytes increased
Special stains	PAS Acid phosphatase for T-cells	Sudan black Peroxidase Esterase	NAP (peripheral blood)	Tartrate-resistant acid phosphatase for hairy cell leukaemia Reticulin ±		Thionin (trephine)	Reticulin

paired morphologically, and similar pairs are grouped together. There are seven groups allotted A to G.

Each chromosome has four arms: two short and two long, designated p and q respectively. When describing chromosomal changes, plus and minus signs signify added or lost material. Analysis of chromosomal patterns has been aided by the development of chromosomal banding techniques. These techniques permit precise identification of each human chromosome and of segments of these chromosomes. As a result, non-random patterns of chromosomal gains and losses have been identified in leukaemic cells.

Certain chromosome rearrangements, especially specific translocations, are consistently associated with particular types of leukaemia.

- Translocation between chromosomes 9 and 22 [t(9;22)] — chronic granulocytic leukaemia (Philadelphia chromosome).
- t(8;21) — acute myeloblastic leukaemia — M2 in the French–American–British classification (FAB).
- t(15;17) — acute promyelocytic leukaemia — M3 FAB.
- t(8;14) — B-cell malignancies.

The meaning of these consistent translocations is uncertain, but recent work suggests that they occur at break-points close to the site of cellular oncogenes and they may result in changes which induce activation.

Chromosomal abnormalities not only define certain types of leukaemia but they are also important clinical prognostic indicators.

Acute myeloblastic leukaemia. Clonal abnormalities are found in 50% of cases. Patients with only normal metaphases have a better prognosis. The 8;21 translocation is found in 8% and the disease is particularly aggressive when the abnormality is associated with a missing sex chromosome.

Acute lymphoblastic leukaemia. The karyotype is an independent prognostic factor which has a significant influence on survival even when other major risk factors are considered. Overall survival is better in the hyperdiploid and hypodiploid categories and shortest in the pseudodiploid group.

Secondary acute leukaemia. In patients who develop acute leukaemia after previous cytotoxic or radiation therapy, non-random clonal chromosome abnormalities are almost always present.

Philadelphia (Ph) positive acute leukaemia. It was previously regarded that all such cases represented CGL in blast transformation. Many such patients have no evidence of a previous chronic phase and it is now accepted that Ph+ve acute leukaemia may arise *de novo*. Most of the cases are AML, but about 20% of adult cases of ALL are Ph+ve. Response to treatment tends to be poor and survival short.

Chronic granulocytic leukaemia. Between 92 and 96% of patients have the typical Ph,t(9;22). In about 8% variants are present, some of which involve 9, 22, and other chromosomes in complex translocations. The commonest changes are an extra Ph or no. 8 chromosome. In males the Y chromosome is missing in about 9%, a phenomenon recognized in other myeloproliferative disorders. Less than 10% show abnormalities additional to the Ph chromosome in the chronic phase, whereas up to 75% show changes in the acute phase.

Clinical chemistry

Biochemical investigation of the body fluids, in particular serum, is an important adjunct to management of disease states. Multiple analysis of single samples has highlighted patterns of abnormality that affect morbidity and mortality, and as such make clinical chemistry an extension of history and physical examination.

Hypercalcaemia is detectable in up to 35% of myeloma patients at presentation and more rarely in high-grade malignant lymphoma.

Symptoms include:
- Thirst.
- Polyuria.
- Constipation.
- Abdominal pains.
- Lethargy.
- Confusion/coma.

In malignant disease this is usually secondary to bone destruction due to release of 'osteoclast-activating factor' (OAF) by tumour cells. Its development is exacerbated by abnormal renal function, impairment of which may be due to the high calcium load effect on the distal tubule.

Hypocalcaemia may develop is association with hypomagnesaemia during the treatment of acute leukaemia. Causes include:

- Acute tumour lysis which generates phosphate binding of calcium and magnesium.
- Diarrhoea with faecal loss of calcium and magnesium together with malabsorption of vitamin D. This occurs following total body irradiation, cytotoxic drug therapy and treatment with antibiotics.
- Reduced immunoreactive parathormone (PTH). Parathyroid function is affected by a number of factors:

1 Antimicrobial agents, especially aminoglycosides.

2 Cytotoxic drugs including anthracyclines, cytarabine and vinca alkaloids.

3 Hypomagnesaemia which inhibits secretion of PTH. Urinary loss of magnesium is enhanced by secondary hyperaldosteronism resulting from hypovolaemia and hypoalbuminaemia, having the additional effects of reduced end organ response to PTH, diminished response to vitamin D, and decreased ionic bone exchange of calcium and magnesium.

Hyponatraemia is usually not suspected clinically unless routine measurements are undertaken but contributes significantly to morbidity and mortality.

Clinical features of a plasma sodium below 120 mmol/l are:

- Headache.
- Depression and/or personality change.
- Irritability and lack of cooperation.
- Lethargy and drowsiness.
- Anorexia, nausea, and vomiting.
- Cramps and weakness.
- Pseudobulbar palsy.
- Rigidity.
- Diminished reflexes.
- Extensor plantar responses.
- Confusion, coma, fits and death.

Underlying changes are:

- Increased extracellular fluid (ECF) volume without concomitant sodium retention.
- Sodium loss from the ECF without proportional water loss.
- Shift of sodium or water between ECF and intracellular fluid (ICF) volume.

Causative factors are:

- Spurious hyponatraemia — displacement of plasma water by lipid.
- Hyponatraemia due to solute accumulation, as in hyperglycaemia.
- Redistribution ('sick cell syndrome').
- Depletion and dehydration due to vomiting and diarrhoea.
- Dilution — syndrome of inappropriate ADH secretion (SIADH), e.g. intrathoracic or CNS disease, drugs (cyclophosphamide, vincristine, diuretics), Hodgkin's disease, acute myeloid leukaemia, inappropriate intravenous therapy.
- Depletion and dilution, e.g. diuretics in congestive failure.

Hyperkalaemia has been described in Burkitt's lymphoma and ALL following chemotherapy and may result in sudden death. In any tumour with many cells in active proliferation cytotoxics cause rapid tumour lysis with release of intracellular potassium into the plasma.

Spurious hyperkalaemia may be found in extreme leucocytosis or thrombocytosis due to leakage of potassium from the cells after sample collection. This has no clinical significance and inappropriate treatment can be dangerous.

Hypokalaemia often occurs at some stage during the treatment of acute leukaemia due to:

- Renal tubular damage by serum lysozyme (*see below*).
- Urinary loss due to the high sodium load of the antibiotic regimens used.
- SIADH.
- Renal infiltration with tumour.

Hyperuricaemia is particularly prevalent in malignant disease because of:

- Increased uric acid manufacture due to high cell turnover.
- Reduced renal excretion secondary to renal damage which may be due to the disease, treatment, infection or the high uric acid level alone.
- The effect of cytotoxic agents which cause a rapid cell kill followed by uric acid release.

Chronic malignant processes such as CGL lead to gout due to accumulation of crystals in the synovial fluid. Acute processes are more likely to lead to uric acid nephropathy. Rapid rises in plasma levels cause crystal deposition in the kidney. Relatively good renal function is preserved until advanced and widespread changes have occurred.

Uric acid crystals cause:

- Nephrotoxicity.
- Interstitial fibrosis and tubular degeneration.
- Precipitation in the tubular lumen and collecting ducts with urate stones.
- Reduced solubility as the urinary pH fails.

Liver-associated enzymes. The enzymes most useful in detecting release from damaged tissue are widely distributed, so that changes in their levels do not by themselves indicate which tissue is affected. However, as the liver is so richly supplied patterns of response can be used to infer disease processes.

Alanine transaminase (ALT) concentrations are high in liver parenchymal cells, and raised levels invariably indicate liver pathology:

- Damage to as few as 1 in 750 parenchymal cells produces a measurable rise in ALT.

γ-Glutamyl transferase (GGT) is a very sensitive screening test for the presence of hepatobiliary disease but lacks specificity and has little differential diagnostic value in liver disease.

Lactic acid dehydrogenase (LDH)

As this enzyme catalyses the interconversion of lactate and pyruvate it is present in high concentration in many cells. Increased levels have little diagnostic significance unless very high; levels increase if blood is not separated within 30 minutes of venepuncture. High levels are found in:

- Haemolytic anaemia.
- Megaloblastic anaemia.
- Acute leukaemia.
- Any damage to cardiac, cerebral, hepatic or renal tissue.

Alkaline phosphatase (AP)

- Increased osteoblastic activity from any cause raises the activity of alkaline phosphatase.
- Children and adolescents normally have raised serum levels.
- Most pronounced elevations are in diseases which affect the biliary tract.
- Levels may remain normal in hepatic processes.

Four different isoenzymes appear in the serum:

- Placental.
- Intestinal.

- Hepatic.
- Bone.

Differentiation of the last two by isoenzyme analysis is important in malignant disease to confirm possible affected tissue. Placental AP may increase non-specifically in 5–15% of patients with malignant disease.

- Renal alkaline phosphatase rarely appears in the circulation.

Plasma proteins

Albumin. A fall in plasma albumin may be seen following any severe injury or during any serious illness. A reduction of up to 25% is not unusual. Causes include:

- Increased catabolic rate.
- Reduced liver production.
- Sequestration in protein-rich effusions.
- Gastrointestinal loss with malignant infiltration.

Table 3.18 Patterns of abnormality in liver disease.

Disorder	ALT	AST	LDH	GT	Alkaline phosphatase
Acute hepatitis					
viral	+++	+++	++	++	N or +
drugs	++	++	+	++	N or +
Chronic hepatitis	++	++	N or +	++	+
Cirrhosis					
post-hepatitic	N or +	+	N or +	++	N or +
alcoholic					
metabolic					
Cholestasis					
intrahepatic	++	++	N or +	++	++
extrahepatic	+	+	N or +	+++	+++
Malignant infiltration	N or +	+	+	++	+

N = normal; + to +++ = increasing degree of abnormality.

3.13 Tissue diagnostic procedures

Table 3.19 Normal immunoglobulins.

Structure	Molecular weight	Mean serum concentration (g/l)	Distribution intravascular: extravascular	Half-life (days)
IgG monmer	160 000	12	45 : 55	23
IgA dimer	170 000	2.5	40 : 60	6
IgM pentamer	1 000 000	1.0	80 : 20	5

Globulin. Changes in the concentration and proportions of the immunoglobulins in plasma occur in a wide range of diseases. Except in the paraproteinaemias when the change is monoclonal (affecting usually one heavy chain and one light chain), the alteration is polyclonal (affecting a mixture of heavy and light chains). Analysis of the changes by immunoelectrophoresis allows the malignant paraprotein to be identified.

- IgG is present throughout body fluid. Produced in response to soluble toxins, viruses and bacteria, it opsonizes and facilitates removal and destruction of foreign tissue.
- IgA, secreted by mucosal surfaces, is the first line of defence against infectious organisms.
- IgM, macroglobulin, is primarily in the blood compartment. It binds complement, facilitating lysis.
- IgE is important in allergy.
- Bence Jones protein (BJP) is found mainly in the urine of patients with myeloma. In normal subjects the excretion is so small as to be virtually undetectable.

BJP can be detected by heating acidified urine. A precipitate forms below 60 °C which redissolves on further heating. Accurate detection requires immunoelectrophoresis of concentrated urine.

β_2-Microglobulin is the light chain of the HLA antigen on the surface of all nucleated cells, whose turnover is the source of the free substance in blood. It is freely filtered by the kidney and is

3.13 Tissue diagnostic procedures

Table 3.20 Immunoglobulin patterns in disease.

Disorder	IgG	IgA	IgM
Bacterial infections	++	++	++
Chronic viral and protozoal infections; Primary biliary cirrhosis	− or +	+ or −	++
Chronic mucosal inflammation	− or +	++	− or +
Connective tissue disorders	++	− or +	− or +
Uraemia; Chronic lymphocytic leukaemia; Malignant lymphoma	−−	−	−
IgG myeloma	++	−	−
IgA myeloma	−	++	−
Bence Jones protein myeloma	−	−	−
Waldenstrom's macro-globulinaemia	− or +	+ or −	++

Key: ++, increased; + or −, variably affected; −, marginally affected; −−, reduced.

catabolized in the tubules. The concentration rises as the glomerular filtration rate falls, and raised amounts occur in advanced adenocarcinoma, but the relationship is inconstant. Changes in serum concentration do reflect changes of clinical importance in haematological malignancies and are independent of changes in acute phase reactants and ESR.

Estimation of β_2-microglobulin has been used in the management of:

- *CLL*. There is a relationship between β_2-microglobulin and clinical stage, but not peripheral lymphocyte count.

- *Non-Hodgkin's lymphoma*. Higher levels are associated with a poor prognosis.
- *Myeloma*. Concentrations are unrelated to glomerular filtration rate or paraprotein type, but levels do correlate with estimates of tumour mass and are rarely raised in benign gammopathy.
- *Hodgkin's disease*. Concentrations increase with stage, and high concentrations before treatment are related to survival.
- *CNS extension of leukaemia or lymphoma* may be associated with elevated levels in the CSF.

C-reactive protein. An acute phase reactant may be useful in differentiating pyrexia due to infection from other causes in patients with leukaemia undergoing intensive therapy and in sickle cell crisis.

3.14 Imaging techniques

A variety of techniques are now available to produce an image of an organ or structure within the body.

Conventional radiography will in many instances provide adequate data so that further procedures can be planned.

The plain PA chest X-ray supplemented by tomographic and lateral views will highlight the bones, lung parenchyma and mediastinum. This may be all that is necessary in clinical staging of the lymphomas and myeloma. In previously undiagnosed mediastinal masses the differential diagnosis is wide.

A skeletal survey may be performed if bony lesions are suspected, and this should be supplemented by isotope imaging (*see below*).

A plain abdominal X-ray may aid assessment of organ size in the obese patient in whom palpation is difficult, but often this will need to be augmented by the use of computed tomography or ultrasound.

Mediastinal masses

Anterior	Retrosternal thyroid Dermoid Thymic mass Lymphoma Pericardial cyst Aortic aneurysm
Middle	Bronchogenic carcinoma Lymphoma Sarcoidosis Primary tuberculosis Fungal disease
Posterior	Neurogenic tumours Paravertebral tumour extension Paravertebral abscess Aortic aneurysm

Computed tomography (CT). CT differs from conventional radiography in that it primarily produces tissue density measurements and only secondarily is a picture created. It is essentially tomographic, examining the body, a section at a time, in the axial plane. The technique is valuable where organ contour is distorted or where a lesion has a density different from its surroundings. CT can distinguish soft tissues from cysts or fat, but cannot distinguish inflammatory from malignant material.

Patients with suspected malignancy are ideal for such examination. The site of origin of a mass may be determined, assisting more definitive diagnostic procedures. Accurate staging, which is important in the malignant lymphomas, is aided; lesions as small as 3 mm may be detected in the lungs, and unsuspected disease in vertebral bodies may be seen. Retroperitoneal node masses, particularly those above L3 which are difficult to detect by other techniques, may be identified. CT scanning, however, does not demonstrate internal architecture, size being the only criterion for abnormality. Confusion may therefore arise in that glands enlarged by reactive hyperplasia and nodular involvement of a normal-sized gland will be misclassified. Similarly, diffuse involvement of organs cannot be demonstrated, and so staging laparatomy with splenectomy remains a part of assessment in the lymphomas. Head scanning is extremely useful in the assessment of intracranial lesions, especially:

- Malignant infiltration of the brain.
- Haemorrhage in the haemostatic disorders.
- Infection.

Magnetic resonance imaging (MRI). This is the newest technique in radiology but does not use ionizing radiation. It depends on magnetic fields and radiofrequency pulses to produce images. These images are very similar to those produced by CT.

Ultrasonography uses non-ionizing radiation and has made a considerable impact over the last two decades in practical obstetrics. It has also been widely used in imaging organs such as liver, pancreas, kidney and spleen. The technique is dependent on an experienced operator and careful patient preparation and is affected by fat or gas so that a picture may not be obtained. With this technique an unacceptable number of false-negative and false-positive results may occur, and it has little place alone in diagnostic oncology. In diagnostic procedures it should usually be combined with an isotope imaging technique, but its main value is that it can monitor organ size in a quick, non-invasive way. It is valuable in the diagnosis of venous thrombosis and of intra-abdominal haemorrhage in haemostatic disorders.

Isotope imaging provides information that is complementary to the other techniques, as it provides a more functional assessment of the structures rather than purely anatomical images. In oncology its place has been largely taken over by computed tomography. It remains useful in metastatic bone disease, but since many benign conditions produce a similar appearance the standard radiograph and the isotope image should be considered together.

A recent development has been the labelling of white cells using indium-111 which when injected into the patient may localize areas of infection. This is a specialized technique and requires further evaluation.

Diagnostic imaging — preferential techniques

CT scanning	Brain
	Eye and orbit
	Mediastinum
	Chest wall
	Lymph nodes
	Retroperitoneal space
	Pelvis
MRI	Brain
	posterior fossa
	spinal cord
	Muscle
	Liver
	Kidney
Ultrasound	Eye and orbit
	Cardiac valves
	Pelvis
	Liver, gall bladder, biliary tree
	Breasts
Radionuclide imaging	Brain
	Lymphatics
	Bones including marrow
	Venous circulation
	Urogenital tract
	Adrenals

4 Haematological practice

4.1 Haematinics, anaemia and iron overload

Deficiencies of iron, vitamin B_{12} and folic acid lead directly to anaemia in man, but other forms of anaemia may be associated with abnormalities in the way the body deals with these or other chemicals. An excess of iron can accumulate in the body and cause tissue damage.

Iron deficiency

This is due either to a reduced intake or to increased loss of body iron. The main causes are:

- Lack of iron in the diet, especially haemoglobin iron.
- Failure to absorb iron, usually due to achlorhydria, gastric surgery or malabsorption.
- Menorrhagia.
- Childbirth.
- Gastrointestinal bleeding.
- Bleeding from the renal tract.

Other potential sources of iron loss are:

- Chelation within the bowel by drugs such as tetracycline or substances such as phytates.
- Loss due to rare disorders such as paroxysmal nocturnal haemoglobinuria and pulmonary haemosiderosis.
- Skin loss in exfoliative dermatitis.

Iron deficiency often develops slowly, and symptoms may be minimal even at quite low haemoglobin levels. Typically the patient complains of:

- Tiredness.
- Shortness of breath

and is pale on examination of the conjunctivae. In addition there may be:

- Angular cheilosis — splitting of the corner of the mouth.
- Glossitis.
- Koilonychia — concave finger nails which are brittle.

The Plummer–Vinson or Paterson–Kelly syndrome, which is a combination of iron deficiency and a post-cricoid web with dysphagia, is *extremely* rare but may predisopose to carcinoma of the oesophagus.

The peripheral blood shows a hypochromic microcytic picture which may be masked by the anaemia of chronic disease if there is an underlying inflammatory or neoplastic cause. The most useful parameter apart from the haemoglobin concentration is the MCV, which is usually below 70 fl. The platelet count may be increased due to bleeding or inflammatory stimulation of the bone marrow.

Diagnosis

This is usually fairly obvious, but should be confirmed by the finding of:

- Low iron and elevated TIBC.
- Serum ferritin — levels below 15 μg/l are diagnostic. Inflammatory conditions may bring the ferritin concentration into the normal range despite the presence of iron deficiency.

There is rarely any need to examine the bone marrow for the diagnosis of iron deficiency alone.

It is important to look for the underlying cause of the anaemia in all cases. This requires clinical judgement, and the approach is obviously different when treating a young woman as opposed to an elderly man.

Differential diagnosis

Laboratory aspects are considered in detail on p. 56. Other likely causes of hypochromic microcytic anaemia are:

- β-Thalassaemia minor.
- α-Thalassaemia.
- Anaemia of chronic disease.
- Sideroblastic anaemia.

Thalassaemia can usually be excluded by haemoglobin electrophoresis and family studies. It should be remembered that thalassaemia minor and iron deficiency can coexist. If there is evidence of iron deficiency then this should be treated and the patient restudied when iron stores have been replenished. The anaemia of chronic disease is usually normocytic, the MCV rarely falling below 70 fl, and the chemical features are characteristic. Patients with sideroblastic anaemia are often elderly, the spleen may be palpable, there is evidence of iron overload and the anaemia may not be very hypochromic.

Treatment

It is rarely necessary to transfuse patients with iron deficiency. If a transfusion is *essential, small* volumes of packed cells should be given *slowly*. Initial treatment should be:

- Ferrous sulphate 200 mg three times a day after food. This provides 180 mg of elemental iron daily. Treatment should continue until three months after the haemoglobin concentration has returned to normal as long as the cause of the initial deficiency has been dealt with.

When patients complain of side-effects such as:

- Constipation.
- Nausea.
- Abdominal pain.
- Diarrhoea.

these are usually due to the iron itself. Reduction in dose is likely to relieve the symptoms but will also reduce the effectiveness of the treatment. An alternative is to use ferrous fumarate or gluconate which may be better tolerated at the same elemental dose, and a liquid form of ferrous fumarate is available, the dose being 10 ml twice daily. Patients quite frequently complain that they do not like or simply do not take the tablets prescribed, and then:

- Ferrograd once daily before food is worth trying as this provides 105 mg of elemental iron in a slow-release form.

For patients who take their tablets regularly and have some gastrointestinal reason for poor absorption, ferrous succinate with added succinic acid may be helpful before accepting the need for parenteral therapy.

4 Haematological practice

4.1 Haematinics, anaemia and iron overload

All iron preparations should be locked away out of the reach of children. Iron poisoning can be fatal.

Parenteral iron. This should be avoided whenever possible. It does not produce a more rapid rise in haemoglobin concentration than oral therapy and is not without risk. The indications are:

- Inability to tolerate oral iron.
- Refusal to take oral iron.
- Treatment of iron deficiency in patients with inflammatory bowel disease.
- Circumstances in which there is no time to observe the effect of the oral iron.

The last indication refers almost exclusively to obstetric practice, where women sometimes present with severe iron deficiency late in pregnancy. Compliance is often poor in this group, and the use of parenteral iron after proper investigation is justifiable. Oral iron should be stopped before beginning treatment.

Iron sorbitol citrate. The daily dose is 1.5 mg iron per kg body weight up to a maximum of 100 mg per injection. The number of injections required can be derived from Table 4.1

Table 4.1

Hb (g/dl)	5.0	6.0	7.0	8.0	9.0	10.0
No. of injections	24	22	20	17	14	12

Deep intramuscular injection via a Z-needle track is used. A substantial quantity of the administered iron is excreted via the kidney and may exacerbate urinary tract infections.

Iron dextran. This may be given intramuscularly but is more commonly used intravenously as a total dose infusion (TDI). It is particularly popular in obstetric practice. The dose is calculated according to the manufacturer's instructions, taking into account the weight of the patient and the haemoglobin concentration. The usual TDI is between 1 and 2 g, which is diluted in 500 ml of normal saline or 5% dextrose for each 1 g infused. The infusion rate should not exceed five drops per minute for the first 10 minutes, but if this test dose is well tolerated the rate may then be increased to 45–60 drops per minute. An antihistamine may be given before starting the infusion, which should be immediately stopped in the event of a reaction.

Iron dextran is not suitable for patients with a definite history of allergy or asthma, and should not be given to patients with rheumatoid arthritis as it can make their symptoms worse. Less important side-effects include flushing, fever, nausea, lymphadenopathy and local phlebitis.

Vitamin B_{12} deficiency

Body stores of vitamin B_{12} last about three years in man so that only long-standing failure to absorb the vitamin will lead to deficiency. Important causes are:

- Pernicious anaemia.
- Post-gastrectomy failure of intrinsic factor production.
- Disease of the terminal ileum.
- Dietary deficiency (especially vegans).

Less commonly are seen:

- Congenital failure to make intrinsic factor (juvenile pernicious anaemia).
- Overgrowth of B_{12}-consuming bacteria in blind loops of bowel or other bowel abnormalities.
- The vitamin B_{12}-dependent fish tapeworm (*Diphyllobothrium latum*) found in Scandinavia and Japan.
- Transcobalamin II deficiency in which serum vitamin B_{12} is normal but there is a lack of the vitamin at a tissue level and the condition presents in infancy.

4 Haematological practice

4.1 Haematinics, anaemia and iron overload

Pernicious anaemia (PA)

PA is a specific autoimmune disorder of the stomach in which a failure to produce Castle's intrinsic factor (IF) results in malabsorption of vitamin B_{12}.

Patients are usually elderly, and the incidence in Northern Europe may be as high as 2% in people in the eighth decade of life. Very rarely the disease may occur in young adults. There is an association with blood group A, and other family members may be affected. Clinical presentation is often insidious, and diagnosis may be delayed until the haemoglobin concentration has fallen to 3 or 4 g/dl. The main clinical findings are:

- Lethargy and malaise.
- Dyspnoea.
- Soreness of the mouth.
- Diarrhoea.
- Pins and needles.
- A curious lemon yellow pallor.
- A smooth, raw tongue.

In addition, about 10% of patients may have a palpable spleen or show evidence of peripheral neuropathy or subacute combined degeneration of the cord (SACD). Clinical associations include:

- Autoimmune thyroiditis.
- Adrenal failure.
- Vitiligo.
- Hypoparathyroidism.
- Hypogammaglobulinaemia.
- Diabetes mellitus.
- Rheumatoid arthritis and keratoconjuctivitis sicca.

The peripheral blood is macrocytic (MCV > 100 fl) and there may be occasional circulating megaloblasts. Leucopenia with hypersegmented neutrophils is common, and thrombocytopenia can occur. The bone marrow is grossly hypercellular and megaloblastic with abnormal granulopoiesis and giant metamyelocytes. Iron is increased in erythroblasts which are sometimes PAS-positive. These features are also seen in the other types of vitamin B_{12} deficiency and megaloblastic anaemia.

Diagnosis

The clinical presentation is often very suggestive unless macrocytosis is an incidental finding. Confirmation is by:

- Serum B_{12} and folate assays.
- Characteristic changes on the B_{12} absorption test (*see* p. 60) which should be performed after treatment.

It is also worth looking for:

- Parietal and intrinsic factor antibodies.

Management

- Do not transfuse patients with PA unless it is *absolutely* necessary. If the transfusion is essential only small volumes of packed cells should be given, very slowly, preferably by exchange transfusion.
- Vitamin B_{12} should be given as hydroxocobalamin 1000 μg intramuscularly daily for three or four days, but the intravenous route can be used if thrombocytopenia is profound. Serum potassium may fall during the early part of treatment. Maintenance therapy is 1000 μg at two-monthly intervals for life.

Although there is an increased incidence of carcinoma of the stomach in PA, it is not usually practicable to search for this complication regularly, but patients should be followed for life by their general practitioner with hospital support if required.

- If the diagnosis is not entirely clear folic acid may be given at the same time as vitamin B_{12}, but folic acid should never be given by itself to patients who may have vitamin B_{12} deficiency.

Post-gastrectomy anaemia

Patients who have had a gastrectomy are sometimes not followed very carefully and may present with fully developed vitamin B_{12} deficiency and SACD, often complicated by iron and folic acid deficiency. Vitamin B_{12} absorption studies give similar results to those of PA, and management is essentially the same as for that condition.

Disease of the terminal ileum

Pathology must be extensive and long-standing to cause vitamin B_{12} deficiency, and the picture is often complicated by other haematinic deficiencies and other causes of anaemia. The most important conditions in this group are:

- Inflammatory bowel disease (Crohn's disease and ulcerative colitis).
- Malabsorption due to gluten-induced enteropathy or tropical sprue.
- Ileal resection and by-pass procedures.

In addition, a congenital failure to absorb vitamin B_{12} at the terminal ileum has been described. Vitamin B_{12} supplements only play a small part in the management of these disorders.

Dietary deficiency

It is necessary to be a strict vegetarian to become deficient in vitamin B_{12}, and most patients seen with this problem are of Asian or Asian–African origin. Anaemia is not necessarily severe and, although macrocytosis is the rule, associated iron deficiency and/or haemoglobinopathy may bring the MCV into the normal range.

- Deficiency of iron and vitamin D is also very common in this group.
- Dietary deficiency of vitamin B_{12} is a reversible cause of infertility.

Investigation reveals no abnormality of vitamin B_{12} absorption, and the most convenient treatment is with small daily doses of oral cyanocobalamin, though this is no longer available under the National Health Service.

Parenteral hydroxocobalamin may be used if desired.

Subacute combined degeneration of the cord (SACD)

Neurological abnormalities arise as a result of vitamin B_{12} deficiency, but probably not in folic acid deficiency. The most common abnormality is:

- Symmetrical peripheral neuropathy.

but more serious is SACD in which there is damage to:

- Corticospinal tracts.
- Dorsal columns.

The precise neurological signs are a variable mixture of these three abnormalities. While treatment will arrest neurological deterioration, cord damage is largely irreversible.

- Treatment of vitamin B_{12} deficiency with folic acid alone may worsen neurological signs.

Folic acid deficiency

Although there is enough folic acid in normal stores to last 12 weeks in a healthy person, it is possible to become deficient much more quickly than this when the rate of utilization is increased. Folic acid deficiency is due to:

- Dietary deficiency, which may arise from an absolute deficiency of vegetables and fruit in the diet or excessive cooking of folate-rich foods (alcoholics are often affected).
- Malabsorption from any cause, especially gluten-induced enteropathy.
- Phenytoin therapy.

and the conditions associated with increased folate demand such as:

- Pregnancy.
- Haemolytic anaemia, including haemoglobinopathy.
- Myeloproliferative disorders and haematological malignancies.
- Severe illness, particularly in patients in intensive care wards who are being fed intravenously with alcohol. Patients undergoing renal dialysis may require folate supplements.

It is possible to induce effective folic acid deficiency with dihydrofolate reductase inhibitors such as methotrexate, pyrimethamine, and trimethoprim, and congenital deficiency of dihydrofolate reductase has been described. The peripheral blood and bone marrow are usually indistinguishable from those found in vitamin B_{12}

deficiency, but if folic acid deficiency occurs very suddenly there may be marked leucopenia and thrombocytopenia with little macrocytosis. The bone marrow must then be examined to make the diagnosis.

Diagnosis
Red cell folate measurement in the untransfused patient more accurately reflects folate status than serum levels.

Management
Oral folic acid 5 mg daily is satisfactory for most patients and may be given prophylactically to patients at high risk of deficiency. A parenteral preparation is available for patients who cannot take the vitamin by mouth. Folinic acid is available to treat those who have been given folate antagonists.

Anaemia of pregnancy (for a fuller discussion *see* p. 295).
The haemoglobin concentration falls physiologically in pregnancy, but many women are truly anaemic at this time. Thus

- Iron deficiency.
- Folic acid deficiency.
- Infection or other illness.
- β-Thalassaemia minor or α-thalassaemia.
- Vitamin B_{12} deficiency.

are likely to interact and precise diagnosis may be difficult. Useful investigations include:

- Careful examination of the peripheral blood.
- Iron and TIBC with serum ferritin.
- Serum folate, red cell folate, and vitamin B_{12}.
- Haemoglobin electrophoresis.
- Tests for haemolysis and infection if indicated.

If a haemoglobinopathy is suspected or confirmed then the family studies must include the husband so that appropriate genetic counselling can be offered.

- In practice a combined iron and folic acid preparation such as

Ferrograd-folic once daily provides 105 mg elemental iron and 350 μg of folic acid and will prevent much anaemia of pregnancy in selected cases.

Oral iron treatment should be tried for iron deficiency when possible, but total dose infusion may be permissible when time is short and the diagnosis is certain. Only when the haemoglobin concentration drops below about 7 g/dl should blood transfusion be considered.

Other causes of macrocytosis and megaloblastosis

Occasionally patients are seen with macrocytosis and/or megaloblastic anaemia which is not due to and does not respond to haematinic therapy. The important causes of this problem are listed in Table 4.2.

Table 4.2

Macrocytosis alone	Macrocytosis and megaloblastosis
Alcoholism	
Liver disease	
Haemolysis	
Reticulocytosis	
Hypothyroidism	
Sideroblastosis	Sideroblastosis
Hypoplasia	Hypoplasia
Preleukaemia	Preleukaemia
	Cytotoxics
	Erythroleukaemia
	Orotic aciduria
	Lesch–Nyhan syndrome

Ascorbic acid

Vitamin C deficiency does not, of itself, cause anaemia, although patients with scurvy are often anaemic. It helps maintain iron in the ferrous state when given by mouth and thereby aids iron absorption. It may be useful for this purpose in achlorhydria. In addition, ascorbic acid increases mobilization of iron in patients with iron overload and has been used to increase iron loss during chelation therapy despite the slight theoretical risk of increasing tissue iron damage during mobilization.

Pyridoxine (vitamin B_6)

Pyridoxine deficiency does not cause anaemia, but pharmacological doses are sometimes helpful in the management of sideroblastic anaemia.

Thiamine

Thiamine-responsive anaemia has occasionally been reported, but thiamine-deficient patients usually have other reasons to be anaemic.

Anaemia of chronic disease

Any significant illness can cause this form of anaemia, particularly:

- Neoplasia.
- Inflammatory and connective tissue disorders.
- Infection.
- Renal disease.

Although the anaemia is typically normocytic and normochromic, microcytosis and hypochromia may occur, but the MCV rarely falls below 70 fl. The distinction from haematinic deficiency is based on:

- The clinical finding of an underlying disease.
- Low plasma iron and TIBC with normal ferritin.
- Normal bone marrow iron stores.
- The lack of response to haematinics, if given.

The anaemia is due to poor utilization of iron together with ineffective erythropoiesis. It is often complicated by haematinic deficiency, blood loss, bone marrow failure or infiltration, hypersplenism, and lack of erythropoietin, and will only respond to the treatment of the underlying condition.

Sideroblastic anaemias

The common theme of the sideroblastic anaemias is a failure to incorporate iron into haem within the erythroblast due to a metabolic defect. Iron accumulates within mitochrondria, and since these are arranged around the nucleus the iron granules appear as rings giving rise to the term 'ring sideroblast'. Unless the spleen has been removed, siderotic granules do not appear in mature red cells in the peripheral blood.

Patients have the symptoms of anaemia, and the spleen may be palpable, but other clinical features depend on the underlying cause and the course of the condition.

- The peripheral blood is typically 'dimorphic' with some well-haemoglobinized and some poorly haemoglobinized cells.
- Both hypochromic microcytic and macrocytic morphology are seen.
- The bone marrow may show megalobastosis or dyserythropoiesis as well as the ring sideroblasts.
- Iron overload occurs with saturated iron binding capacity, raised serum ferritin, and increased bone marrow iron.

In the later stages of the disease there is often evidence of tissue iron damage, especially to the liver, and hepatic biopsy may be helpful to assess this in some cases.

Congenital sideroblastic anaemia

This is often X-linked so boys are more commonly affected than girls. Such patients are sometimes transfusion-dependent but may respond to pharmacological doses of pyridoxine (300 mg daily) and folic acid supplements.

- Iron overload may be prevented by venesection if a reasonable haemoglobin concentration can be maintained.
- Regular chelation with desferrioxamine should be considered if this is not possible. Occasionally it may be worth combining venesection and chelation, depending on the degree of iron overload and the commitment of patient and physician to long-term therapy. The cost of this approach is considerable.

Primary acquired sideroblastic anaemia

The majority of patients are middle-aged or elderly without any clear underlying disorder. The principles of management are the same as for congenital disease, but it is difficult for elderly patients to undertake demanding chelation therapy and this is usually unnecessary. Life expectancy in this group is often limited by age and general condition rather than iron overload, and some go on to develop acute leukaemia.

Secondary acquired sideroblastic anaemia

Reversible causes are:

- Antituberculous therapy.
- Alcohol.
- Chloramphenicol.
- Lead poisoning.
- Malnutrition.

and the treatment is removal of the cause.

Haematological causes are:

- Myeloma.
- Leukaemia.
- Myeloproliferative disease.

in which sideroblastosis indicates a probably irreversible stem cell defect.

General medical causes include:

- Carcinoma.
- Collagen vascular disease including rheumatoid arthritis.
- Renal failure.

in which the pathogenesis is uncertain and the prognosis is that of the underlying disorder complicated by the sideroblastosis.

Iron overload

Iron absorption is controlled by:

- Body iron stores.
- The rate of erythropoiesis.

which affect the small bowel absorption mechanism. Haemochromatosis has been associated with HLA type but the mechanism is uncertain. Iron overload can result from conditions shown in Table 4.3.

4.1 Haematinics, anaemia and iron overload

Table 4.3 Causes of iron overload.

Cause	Examples
Failure to control absorption	Haemochromatosis Beer brewed in iron pots
Increased rate of erythropoiesis	Haemolytic anaemia, especially thalassaemia major
Regular blood transfusion	Thalassaemia major Aplastic anaemia Sideroblastic anaemia

Iron causes toxic damage as shown in Table 4.4 Death may occur from hepatic or cardiac failure.

Table 4.4 Consequences of iron overload.

Organ	Consequences
Liver	Cirrhosis, hepatoma
Heart	Cardiomyopathy
Pancreas	Diabetes mellitus
Other endocrine organs	Failure of sexual function or development Hypothyroidism
Multifactorial or unknown cause	Pigmentation Arthralgia

The plasma iron is raised and the iron binding capacity is saturated. Serum ferritin is very high and is a useful simple guide to the degree of iron overload. Liver biopsy with iron quantitation has the advantage that tissue damage can be assessed directly. Iron excretion may be measured by quantitating urinary iron after desferrioxamine injection, and this can be useful in planning treatment. If venesection is possible and the volume of blood removed is carefully measured then, when iron stores are exhausted, the original degree of iron overload is known.

Management

- Venesection is the most effective and economic form of treatment if it is possible.
- Chelation with desferrioxamine is considered in detail on p. 165.
- The general medical effects of iron overload are managed in the usual way.

4.2 Pancytopenia

A reduction in all the cellular elements in the peripheral blood can arise from the causes shown in Table 4.5.

Table 4.5 Causes of pancytopenia.

Cause	Examples
Metabolic failure of maturation	Megaloblastic anaemia
Stem cell failure	Aplastic anaemia Paroxysmal nocturnal haemoglobinuria
Bone marrow infiltration	Leukaemia, lymphoma and myeloma Carcinoma Myelofibrosis Granulomas Storage disorders Marble bone disease
Peripheral destruction	Hypersplenism Overwhelming infection

Frequently there is more than one cause contributing to pancytopenia in a particular patient.

- Megaloblastic anaemia is placed first because it is so easily reversible with appropriate therapy, but it will not be considered further here (*see* p. 127).

Aplastic anaemia

In the majority of cases no cause for aplastic anaemia can be demonstrated though autoimmune mechanisms may be responsible. Important causes are:

4.2 Pancytopenia

- Toxic damage by — irradiation.
  — chemicals, especially benzene.
  — cytotoxic drugs.
- Direct or idiosyncratic damage by non-cytotoxic drugs.
- Infection — especially viral hepatitis.
- Pregnancy.
- Paroxysmal nocturnal haemoglobinuria (PNH) (*see* p. 177).
- Congenital predisposition (Fanconi's anaemia).

The most important drugs associated with aplasia are shown below, with the exception of those which are directly cytotoxic.

- Antibiotics
  - chloramphenicol
  - sulphonamides
  - cotrimoxazole
- Antiepileptics
  - phenytoin
  - barbiturates
- Anti-inflammatory
  - most non-steroidal anti-inflammatories, especially phenylbutazone
  - penicillamine
  - gold
  - colchicine
- Antithyroid
  - carbimazole
  - thiouracil
- Anti-ulcer
  - cimetidine
- Antigout
  - allopurinol
- Cardiovascular
  - quinidine
  - captopril

- Diuretics
  - thiazides
- Antituberculous drugs
  - isoniazid
  - PAS
- Antimalarials
  - quinine
  - mepacrine
  - pyrimethamine
- Oral hypoglycaemics
  - tolbutamide
  - chlorpropramide
- Tranquillizers
  - phenothiazines.

This list is in no sense complete, and an exhaustive drug history should be taken from any patient with aplastic anaemia. Whatever the reason for aplasia patients present with the clinical features of bone marrow failure, which are:

- Haemorrhage, especially from mucous membranes.
- Purpura
- Anaemia.
- Infection.

The spleen may be slightly enlarged.

Laboratory diagnosis

Bone marrow aspiration and trephine biopsy are essential, but aspiration may yield little material. The major feature is of markedly reduced cellularity with preservation of marrow architecture, the majority of the sample consisting of bony trabeculae and fat spaces. There may be a significant population of lymphoid cells, and occasional islands of surviving haemopoietic tissue are not uncommon.

The sucrose lysis test for PNH should be performed before

transfusion, and it is worth measuring haemoglobin F. Bone marrow culture and lymphocyte phenotype studies may be valuable.

Management

Severe aplastic anaemia is a very serious disease with a median survival as short as six months with conventional treatment. In order to select patients for the most appropriate treatment, severe aplasia is defined as:

- Neutrophil count below 0.5×10^9/l.
- Platelet count below 20×10^9/l.
- Reticulocyte count below 10×10^9/l.
- Myeloid cells below 20% of bone marrow cells,

and patients under the age of 40 satisfying these criteria should be considered for bone marrow transplantation at diagnosis. Ideally a fully HLA-compatible sibling donor should be selected, but as techniques improve the use of parents and unrelated matched donors is worth considering. In patients who are being considered for bone marrow transplantation it is important to avoid unnecessary sensitization to blood group antigens if at all possible.

This subject is considered in more detail on p. 206 for leukaemia. Up to 50% of patients treated in this way may survive for an indefinite period and may be cured. The results are more favourable in those transplanted early in the course of their disease. For those who are not suitable for transplantation conventional treatment can be offered. This consists of:

- Corticosteroids. These have been given in small, large or very large doses.
- Anabolic steroids such as oxymethalone in doses up to 5 mg/kg/day.
- Antilymphocyte globulin (ALG) as an immunosuppressive agent.
- Cytotoxic agents such as cyclophosphamide have also been given as an immunosuppressant.

It may take three months or more to respond to conventional therapy, but spontaneous recovery may occur and evaluation is difficult. Some patients treated by transplantation have had recovery of their own bone marrow, adding weight to the theory that many cases of aplastic anaemia are immune-mediated.

Support therapy (*see* p. 195 for a fuller account)
Whatever method of treatment is chosen, careful support is essential in the management of bone marrow failure. Depending on the clinical severity this may include:

- Reverse barrier nursing.
- Sterile food.
- Venous access via an intra-atrial catheter.
- Regular microbiological sampling and consultation.
- Prophylactic non-absorbable antibiotics and antifungal agents.
- Immediate treatment of systemic infection.
- Transfusion of leucocyte-poor red cells.
- Platelet concentrates.
- Granulocyte infusions are rarely indicated, but it should be remembered that following immunosuppressant therapy cellular blood products must be irradiated.

NB It can be seen from the above that the management of aplastic anaemia, especially in young people, is best conducted by, or in collaboration with, a large centre.

Congenital aplasia
The best-known form of congenital aplasia is Fanconi's anaemia, which is associated with congenital malformations such as:

- Deformities of the wrist and hand, especially of the thumb and radius.
- Microcephaly and mental retardation.
- Skin pigmentation.
- Short stature and hypogonadism.
- Renal abnormalities.

Inheritance is autosomal recessive, and presentation of the aplasia is often delayed until 5–10 years of age. There is often an abnormal karyotype and raised HbF level, and the condition may terminate in acute leukaemia.

Fanconi's anaemia has some features in common with:

- Congenital thrombocytopenia with absent radius.
- Dyskeratosis congenita — an X-linked disorder in which there is hyperpigmentation, a bizarre dyskeratosis of the skin and nails, hypoplasia and an increased risk of carcinoma.

Bone marrow transplantation is the treatment of choice for Fanconi's anaemia if an unaffected HLA-compatible donor is available.

Red cell aplasia

This rare condition is found:

- In the congenital Diamond–Blackfan syndrome.
- In patients with thymoma sometimes associated with myasthenia gravis and probably mediated by T-suppressor cells.
- As a reversible complication of chronic haemolytic anaemia, possibly related to folic acid deficiency or parvovirus infection.

Bone marrow infiltration

The characteristic peripheral blood finding is leucoerythroblastic anaemia, and pancytopenia may not be profound; indeed the white cell count may be elevated even when the haemoglobin and platelet count are reduced.

The diagnosis is made by bone marrow trephine, and it can be valuable to biopsy at more than one site. The exact point for biopsy is sometimes indicated by radiological or radioisotopic abnormalities. It is essential to stain the trephine sample for reticulin.

Points to remember:

- Myeloma can be patchy, and a single negative biopsy is not conclusive.
- Carcinoma within the bone marrow usually arises from the breast, prostate, or lung. Metastases from the bowel and thyroid are not uncommon.
- Myelofibrosis and granuloma formation are non-specific. The

possibility of underlying lymphoma or tuberculosis should be considered.

• A careful search of the trephine under the low power may be necessary to make the diagnosis of a storage disorder.

Hypersplenism

When the spleen enlarges, for whatever reason, peripheral blood cells are liable to be trapped, pooled and sometimes destroyed within its substance. The consequence is pancytopenia with a normal or hyperplastic bone marrow, the pancytopenia often responding to splenectomy. In addition the spleen may enlarge in haematological disorders in which the bone marrow is abnormal and then contributes to the existing clinical problem. Splenectomy is, again, potentially helpful.

Disorders associated with splenic enlargement and pancytopenia include:

• All forms of haemolysis, especially thalassaemia major, hereditary spherocytosis and autoimmune haemolytic anaemia.
• Malignant lymphomas, especially hairy cell leukaemia.
• Myeloproliferative disorders, especially myelofibrosis.
• Collagen vascular disease, especially Felty's syndrome in rheumatoid arthritis.
• Portal hypertension due to cirrhosis, portal vein thrombosis and hepatic vein thrombosis.
• Storage disorders such as Gaucher's disease.
• Chronic infections such as malaria.

Management

The bone marrow must be examined first as this may immediately establish the diagnosis. Meanwhile general medical investigations can proceed including a barium swallow to exclude oesophageal varices. Liver biopsy may be desirable but is often prevented by thrombocytopenia unless transjugular biopsy is available.

Splenoportography can be helpful where portal vein thrombosis is suspected. Radioactive labelling of red cells with ^{51}Cr and of transferrin with ^{59}Fe can be used to demonstrate the sites of red cell destruction and production respectively, but even when these investigations have been performed the final decision on splenectomy is often a clinical one. Frequently the spleen is removed for reasons other than pancytopenia, but conditions in which this complication is often treated by splenectomy are:

- Thalassaemia major.
- Hairy cell leukaemia.
- Myelofibrosis.
- Felty's syndrome.

Removal of the spleen predisposes to overwhelming infection, particularly by pneumococci, in young people. Pneumococcal vaccine with prophylactic penicillin can be used to reduce this risk.

4.3 The haemolytic anaemias

Haemolysis is defined as a reduction in the red cell life-span to below the normal value of 120 days. It is rarely necessary to measure red cell survival as the diagnosis can usually be made from the clinical state and by simple laboratory observations. These are discussed in detail in Section 3.7 but are summarized below.

- Anaemia, which implies that the haemolysis is uncompensated.
- Red cell morphology.
- Reticulocytosis.
- Jaundice, rarely above 50 μmol/l (unconjugated).
- Raised lactic acid dehydrogenase.
- Increased urobilinogen excretion.
- Decreased haptoglobin.
- Presence of methaemalbumin, haemoglobinaemia, haemoglobinuria and haemosiderinuria.

History and examination

The clinical picture often gives a clue to the underlying cause of the haemolysis and may suggest which diagnostic tests should be performed (Sections 3.7–3.10), avoiding the need for 'blanket' investigation. Particular attention should be paid to:

- Past medical history of undiagnosed jaundice, especially if exacerbated by infection.
- History of neonatal jaundice.
- Surgical history.
- Family history of jaundice or anaemia.
- Drug ingestion.
- Racial origin.
- Physical signs that may suggest an underlying disorder (in particular systemic lupus erythematosus, chronic lymphocytic leukaemia or lymphoma).

Table 4.6 Broad classification of haemolytic anaemias.

Congenital	Acquired
Red cell membrane	Attack by antibodies (a) warm, allo and auto (b) cold
Red cell metabolism	Direct cell injury (a) traumatic (b) drug-related (c) infection
Haemoglobin (a) structure (b) synthesis and chain balance	Paroxysmal nocturnal haemoglobinuria

Congenital haemolytic anaemia

Red cell membrane defects

Hereditary spherocytosis

Inheritance is autosomal dominant with variable penetrance. Up to 20% will have normal parents on study. There is a prevalence of 1 in 5000.

EVIDENCE OF HAEMOLYTIC STATE

Examine intracorpuscular causes

- Morphology
- Osmotic fragility
- Haemoglobin electrophoresis
  - HbA_2
  - HbF
  - specific abnormality
- Assay for commonest enzymopathies
  - G6PD
  - PK
- Assay for other enzymes
- Family studies

Exclude extracorpuscular causes

- Morphology
- Serology
  - antiglobulin test
- Clotting studies
- Infection
  - bacterial
  - parasitization

Fig. 4.1 Investigation of the patient with haemolytic anaemia.

- The spherocyte is characteristic of the condition and is found in a variety of haemolytic states, particularly autoimmune haemolysis. In the latter condition the direct antiglobulin test is positive.

Clinical features. Anaemia is usually mild and well compensated with a persistent reticulocytosis. Exacerbations may be provoked by pregnancy, intercurrent illness or following anaesthesia when temporary bone marrow depression occurs — aplastic crises. Haemolytic crises due to increased splenic sequestration and megaloblastic crises due to folic acid depletion occur but are less common.

The spleen is usually palpable.

Jaundice is usually mild (<50 μmol/l) but it may present at birth and needs to be differentiated from rhesus haemolytic disease of the newborn and G6PD deficiency.

In the mild forms the condition may not present until later in life.

- Chronic leg ulceration is common, usually over the medial malleolus.
- Pigment gall stones occur in over 50% and often cause symptoms in middle age.
- The increased marrow activity may lead to extramedullary haemopoiesis with local pressure symptoms.

Diagnosis:

- Osmotic fragility is increased and confirms the presence of spherocytes.
- The direct antiglobulin test is negative.
- Family studies are usually positive.

Treatment:

- Folic acid supplements are given.
- Splenectomy largely prevents haemolysis and arrests further pigment stone formation.
- Before splenectomy polyvalent pneumococcal vaccine should be given followed by prophylactic maintenance penicillin.
- A cholecystectomy should be considered when splenectomy is performed.
- Blood transfusion should be given as required.

Hereditary elliptocytosis

This is an autosomal disorder of variable penetrance. Elliptocytes are diagnostic but may be mistaken for the pencil-shaped cells seen in iron deficiency. Serum iron measurements are essential. Some families show a genetic linkage between elliptocytosis and certain Rh groups. Haemolysis is variable and may be completely absent. Osmotic fragility studies and the autohaemolysis tests are normal. If the condition is symptomatic splenectomy usually corrects the haemolysis.

Hereditary stomatocytosis
This is a rare condition with autosomal dominant inheritance characterized by red cells with a slit-like central pallor. Many patients do not have anaemia and symptoms are variable. When haemolysis occurs the spleen is usually palpable and splenectomy is beneficial.
• Stomatocytes may be seen transiently after an acute alcoholic binge.

Diagnosis is made on the peripheral blood appearances, signs of haemolysis and family studies.

Spur cell haemolytic anaemia (hereditary acanthocytosis)
Spiculated red cells are found in this autosomal recessive condition. Presentation occurs within the first two years with steatorrhoea due to malabsorption. There is associated ataxia and nystagmus with an atypical retinitis pigmentosa.

Diagnosis is confirmed by the absence of betalipoprotein on lipoprotein electrophoresis.

Acquired acanthocytosis occurs in the terminal stages of liver failure, uraemia, microangiopathic haemolytic anaemia and in association with some neoplasms.

Disorders of red cell metabolism
The metabolism of the red cell was described in Section 3.9. Most congenital enzymopathies affect either the hexose monophosphate shunt or glycolysis (the Embden–Meyerhof pathway). The expression of these enzyme defects probably depends on two unique features of the red cell.
- The long life-span.
- The inability to synthesize protein.

If an enzyme variant is unstable, a deficiency is more likely to be revealed in the red cell than in other tissues. If the enzyme is inactive or particularly unstable, other manifestations may appear in other tissues. Thus there is:
- Leucocyte dysfunction in Mediterranean-type G6PD deficiency.
- Neurological abnormality in cytochrome b reductase deficiency.

- Neurological disorder and cardiac arrhythmia in triosephosphate isomerase deficiency.

With the exception of glucose-6-phosphate dehydrogenase deficiency, symptomatic enzymopathies are rare and, although abnormalities affecting most of the enzyme systems have been described, more common causes of haemolysis should be excluded first. Haemolysis precipitated by drug ingestion is strongly suggestive of an enzyme defect.

Hexose monophosphate shunt

Glucose-6-phosphate dehydrogenase (G6PD)

G6PD is the first enzyme in the hexose monophospate shunt pathway of glucose metabolism. Deficiency reduces the production of NADPH which is necessary for glutathione reduction whose role is to prevent haemoglobin denaturation (by oxidation of sulphydryl groups).

There are over 100 variants of the enzyme of differing clinical significance.

- The normal enzymes are designated types A and B.
- Affected male Negroes have 10–15% residual activity due to an unstable variant of A called A−.
- Reticulocytes in the A− individual have normal activity which declines with cell age. Haemolysis is self-limiting.
- The type seen in the Mediterranean is due to a variant of the B enzyme, B−. Activity is less than 1% and haemolysis may be severe.
- An Oriental type found in South-East Asia is associated with moderately severe deficiency (less than 10% activity).
- Transmission is X-linked.
- The disease is expressed in hemizygous males and homozygous females.
- Heterozygous females have a dimorphic population of red cells due to random deletion of the X chromosome (Lyon hypothesis).

The average G6PD level in affected females is approximately 50%, but individual cells may have low enzyme levels and therefore be liable to haemolysis.

• The condition confers a relative resistance against the malarial parasite, *Plasmodium falciparum*.

Clinical features:

1 Drug-induced haemolysis occurs with all types but is most severe with the Mediterranean and Oriental variants. The Negro type is less severe and haemolysis is often self-limiting as the reticulocytes may contain almost normal levels of activity. Drugs causing haemolysis include:

• Antimalarials — quinine, chloroquine, primaquine.

• Antibacterials — sulphonamides, nitrofurantoin, nalidixic acid, chloramphenicol.

• Antituberculous — para-aminosalicylic acid.

• Antilepromatous — dapsone.

• Analgesics — aspirin, phenacetin.

• Vitamin K.

Haemolysis may be severe enough to cause acute renal failure and death.

2 Favism is characterized by severe haemolysis following ingestion of the uncooked bean of the plant *Vicia fava*. In some patients inhalation of the fava pollen may provoke an attack. This only occurs in the Mediterranean group.

3 Intermittent haemolytic episodes may be provoked by bouts of illness, such as pneumonia, hepatitis or diabetic ketoacidosis.

4 Chronic mild haemolysis occurs with some variants.

5 Neonatal jaundice occurs commonly in the Mediterranean and Oriental types. It can be provoked by the use of vitamin K and must be distinguished from rhesus haemolytic disease of the newborn.

• In all patients the severity of the episode may vary from a clinically inapparent episode to a dramatic and life-threatening intravascular haemolysis associated with loin pain and haemoglobinuria.

Laboratory features:

- Intracellular precipitation of haemoglobin (Heinz bodies), which is particularly prominent following splenectomy.
- Bite cell or blister cells indicate splenic pitting of the inclusion bodies from the cells.
- Reduced G6PD levels are found (discussed in Section 3.9).

Treatment should always include removal of the precipitating drug or agent. Transfusion is rarely required except in neonates.

Embden–Meyerhof pathway

Pyruvate kinase deficiency (PK)

This is the second most common red cell enzyme deficiency and affects the penultimate conversion in the glycolytic pathway. There is impaired production of ATP which is particularly pronounced in stressed red cells leading to calcium gain, potassium and water loss with crenation, and increased cell rigidity. 2,3-DPG levels are also increased with a 'right shift' in the oxygen dissociation curve.

- Deficiency is not simply quantitative and often reflects PK variants with abnormal kinetics.
- Inheritance is autosomal recessive.
- Variants are described with haemolysis in the heterozygous state.
- Deficiency is usually found in North European stock.

Clinical features. Haemolysis can be moderately severe and reticulocytosis can be marked (over 50%). Haemolysis *is not* drug-induced and is spontaneous but may be exacerbated by any physical stress. It usually presents early in life and occasionally as neonatal jaundice.

Splenomegaly is common, as are pigment gall stones.

Laboratory findings. Red cell PK is reduced to less than 20% of normal. 2,3-DPG and other glycolytic metabolites are increased.

Autohaemolysis is increased without correction by glucose but is reduced by ATP.

Treatment. Transfusion may be necessary at times of intense haemolysis, and exchange transfusion is required for the neonate.

Splenectomy may improve the haemolytic state but does not correct it as in hereditary spherocytosis.

Folate supplements are usually necessary.

Disorders of haemoglobin synthesis

Over 300 variants of the molecular structure of the globin chains of haemoglobin have been described, and the majority are clinically insignificant.

Inheritance follows a simple Mendelian pattern. Any child of two heterozygotes has a 1 in 4 chance of being an abnormal homozygote, a 1 in 4 chance of being normal and a 1 in 2 chance of inheriting the heterozygous (usually carrier) state.

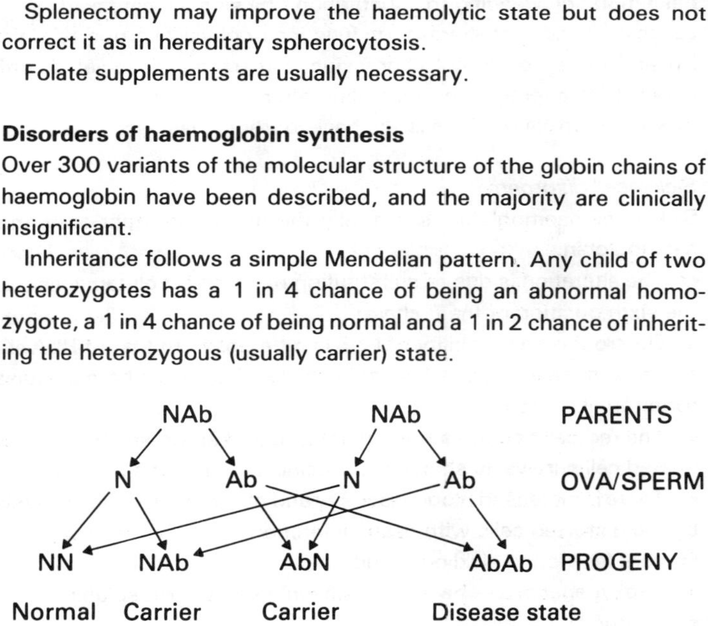

Fig. 4.2 Mendelian inheritance. N = Normal; Ab = abnormal.

Of the two pairs of globin chains the α pair are coded for on chromosome 16 and the β pair on chromosome 11. A defect in the α-chain affects HbA, F and A_2, whereas a defect in β-chain production involves only HbA.

A defect in the β-chain will not present until the production of HbF has died away (at about six months) whereas an abnormality of the α-chain will affect the fetus from conception.

Defects in haemoglobin structure

The vast majority of the structural variants of Hb represent single base mutations leading to substitution of a single amino acid. Most cause no significant alteration in function or physical property of the Hb and have no clinical expression. Others are associated with intracellular aggregation, instability, altered O_2 affinity or methaemoglobin formation. This is the basis of most classifications.

Sickle cell disorders

Sickle cell haemoglobin is clinically the most important abnormal haemoglobin.

- The alteration is due to substitution of valine for glutamic acid at the sixth position of the β-chain.
- Electrophoretic mobility of HbS is different from that of HbA.
- Deoxygenated HbS is less soluble than HbA and the molecules form rod-like 'tactoids'.
- The red cell becomes rigid, deformed and sickle-shaped.
- Red cell survival is shortened causing a haemolytic anaemia.
- There is increased blood viscosity and obstruction of fine vessels by the distorted cells with tissue infarction.

Factors facilitating sickling include:

- Deoxygenation — because of the influence of Hb solubility.
- Acidosis.
- Stasis — because it exacerbates acidosis and reduces oxygen tension.
- Dehydration — which raises the MCHC and blood viscosity, reducing blood flow.
- Temperature — as cold favours stasis and precipitates sickling.

The presence of other haemoglobins, e.g. HbF, may reduce the tendency to sickle.

Incidence
The gene is largely found in Negro populations. The highest carrier rate is in a belt across Central Africa (20%). It is also found in areas to which people from Central Africa have emigrated, especially North, Central and South America, the Caribbean and Europe. It is also found in Greece, the Middle East and in some East Indian tribes.

Sickle cell trait (haemoglobin S)
The carrier is usually healthy, and as each red cell contains only 40% of HbS sickling occurs only under extreme circumstances. Conditions that provoke anoxia should be avoided.

- High-altitude flying in unpressurized aircraft.
- Deep sea diving.
- Surgery involving the use of a tourniquet or if deoxygenation is likely.

Clinical features. In the normal state carriers are asymptomatic and should have no restrictions on their lifestyle.

Respiratory infections, paticularly if the patient becomes dehydrated, may lead to sickling.

Haematuria is common and is thought to be due to renal papillary necrosis secondary to sickling in the acidotic environment of the renal medulla.

- Genetic counselling should be offered to all at-risk mothers.
- Prenatal diagnosis is feasible if both partners carry the trait.
- Post-natal diagnosis can be performed at birth.

Diagnosis. The peripheral blood film and indices are completely normal. A screening test with a reducing agent (e.g. sodium metabisulphite) to induce *in vitro* sickling or Hb electrophoresis should be performed on all at-risk individuals.

Sickle cell disease (haemoglobin SS)
Symptoms develop in the latter part of the first year of life as the protective effect of fetal haemoglobin wanes. The patient runs a

'steady state' haemoglobin of 6–8 g/dl with a persistent reticulocytosis of up to 20%. The haemoglobin present is almost exclusively HbS with a little HbF. This steady state is interspersed with crises.

Crises that increase anaemia

1 Haemolytic crises cause a further reduction in Hb. They may follow infection and have been associated with concomitant G6PD deficiency.

2 Aplastic crisis in which marrow activity temporarily ceases is associated with parvovirus infections and may be lethal. Recovery occurs after one week with an intense reticulocytosis.

3 Sequestration crises occur in young children. The spleen greatly enlarges and may hold most of the blood volume.

4 Megaloblastic crises due to superimposed folic acid deficiency may exacerbate the anaemia and are a problem in pregnancy.

Infarctive crises

1 Vaso-occlusive crises are caused by entangled sickle cells and are characterized by severe pain. These occur in any organ in which blood flow may be sluggish — the spleen, bone and penis. The typical painful crisis usually involves the simultaneous occurrence of pain in multiple areas of the body — limbs, lower back, abdomen and chest. Splenomegaly is common in young children but recurrent splenic infarction is so common that the spleen has scarred itself away by the age of five, 'autosplenectomy'.

Priapism is usually due to massive sickling in the corpora cavernosa.

2 Hand–foot syndrome occurs in infancy due to a dactylitis affecting the dorsum of the hands and feet. This is due to medullary infarction.

Other features

1 Osteomyelitis is a common complication, especially due to Salmonellae. It may be difficult to differentiate from bone infarction with a subsequent periosteal reaction.

2 Chronic leg ulceration is common and extremely painful and may require skin grafting.

3 Neurological complications occur with meningitis and infarction, and visual impairment may follow arteriolar occlusion. Vascular proliferation on the retina is often seen. Subsequent vitreous haemorrhage may predispose to retinal detachment.

4 Gall stones due to haem pigment occur in up to half of patients but are usually asymptomatic.

Management. Infarction pain may vary from mild to agonizing, and when severe is often accompanied by constitutional symptoms. It may be difficult to differentiate a precipitating cause from the effects of the vaso-occlusion. Treatment needs to be urgent, adequate and sympathetic, ideally by a physician with an interest in the disease who will follow the patients in a 'sickle clinic'. Treatment of the crisis should include:

- Rehydration.
- Treatment of obvious infection (but consider blind 'broad-spectrum' treatment).
- Adequate analgesia.
- Oxygen therapy, which is often given but is of dubious value.
- Transfusion, usually by exchange. This should be considered only if:

1 Anaemia is severe.
2 Surgery is contemplated.
3 There is priapism.
4 The acute respiratory syndrome is diagnosed.
5 The crisis is prolonged.

- Anti-sickling agents are as yet of unproven value.
- The use of i.v. bicarbonate to correct acidosis, while theoretically sound, is of limited practical value.

Long-term management:

- Early and vigorous treatment of infection.
- Folic acid supplements.

- Avoidance of conditions likely to provoke sickling.
- Prophylactic penicillin and polyvalent pneumococcal vaccine in view of the increased infection risk due to the functional asplenism.
- School work should be encouraged as children may have frequent absences due to crises.
- Social conditions are important as it is now recognized that good conditions and concern for improved public health care directly affect survival.
- Patients who suffer recurrent crises may be offered a period of exchange transfusion, although this is not without long-term risk.
- Contraception — barrier techniques are the method of choice but the progestogen-only pills are not associated with increased thrombosis. Intrauterine devices are associated with increased pelvic inflammatory disease.
- In pregnancy both the mother and the fetus are at risk from the effects of sickling crises, and exchange transfusion should be considered from the beginning of the second trimester (*see* Section 4.9)

Other sickling disorders

Sickle cell disease with hereditary persistence of haemoglobin F (HPHF). Patients with sickle cell disease (HbSS) who also have HPHF have high levels of HbF which reduce the risk of sickling. The disease is mild and the spleen is palpable in up to 50%. The haemoglobin level is normal but Hb electrophoresis demonstrates HbS 80%, HbF 20%, and variable HbA_2 with no HbA.

Haemoglobin SC. There is a combination of HbS and HbC in equal proportions. Anaemia is usually mild and the film shows a mixture of target and sickle cells. Avascular necrosis of the femoral heads and retinal damage are the most important clinical problems but sickle crises are rare. In pregnancy and the puerperium thrombotic episodes occur and may be fatal. Exchange transfusion is usually offered (*see* Secion 4.9). Splenomegaly occurs in most patients.

Haemoglobin S/β-thalassaemia is a combination of HbS and β-thalassaemia trait. The severity of the condition depends on whether the β^0 or β^+ gene has been inherited and therefore whether HbA is produced. In HbS/β^0-thalassaemia no normal adult Hb is produced and the disease is comparable to sickle cell anaemia. The cells are hypochromic and contain HbS, with variable amounts of HbF and HbA_2. In HbS/β^+-thalassaemia there is greater than 50% HbS, but variable amounts of HbA, HbF and HbA_2 are present. The coexistence of α-thalassaemia trait and sickle cell disease results in a comparatively mild clinical condition.

Other haemoglobin structural disorders

Haemoglobin C. HbC is found in West Africa, particularly Ghana, where up to 20% are carriers. There is a substitution of the sixth amino acid of the β-chain of lysine for glutamic acid.

The trait is asymptomatic and the haemoglobin level normal. The disease is often asymptomatic, but splenomegaly occurs and dehydration may provoke haemolysis.

The anaemia is mild with a reticulocytosis of approximately 5%, and the film shows many target cells.

Haemoglobins D and E. These abnormal haemoglobins cause relatively little clinical upset although they are quite common worldwide. Both are β-chain variants and the homozygous disease shows a mild haemolytic anaemia. HbD is most common in North-West India and there are numerous variants; HbE is found in South-East Asia.

Unstable haemoglobins. Mutations that disrupt the tertiary structure of globin result in a haemoglobin molecule that denatures, forming Heinz bodies within the cell. These are aggregates of denatured haemoglobin. Heinz bodies are removed in the spleen and damage the cell membrane leading to premature cell destruction and a haemolytic anaemia. Most are inherited as autosomal dominant.

Haemolysis may be episodic (usually on exposure to oxidant drugs as with Hb Zurich or Hb Köln) or chronic (with variants such as Hb Hammersmith).

Hb electrophoresis may be normal or abnormal. Heinz bodies may only be obvious in splenectomized patients. The unstable Hb may be demonstrated by a variety of stability tests. It is important to avoid oxidant drugs.

Haemoglobins with altered oxygen affinity. Amino acid substitutions may alter the affinity of the molecule for oxygen, thus altering the curve of oxygen dissociation. A useful screening test is the measurement of the P_{50} (*see* p. 71), which is the Po_2 at which Hb is half-saturated with O_2. In man the normal value is 27.0 ± 1.0 mmHg at 37 °C.

1 Increased affinity ('a left shift') — the haemoglobin is incapable of releasing oxyen to the tissue. Relative tissue anoxia stimulates the marrow with production of erythrocytosis. Mutations affect either $\alpha\beta$ contact (Hb Chesapeake) or binding of 2,3-DPG (Hb Rahere), and inheritance is autosomal dominant. Spleen size, WBC and platelets are normal, as is arterial Po_2. In general the lower the P_{50} the higher the Hb, but some variants are unstable (e.g. haemoglobin pocket — Hb Heathrow) and the Hb level may be normal. If the haematocrit is greater than 0.55, venesection should be considered to reduce the cardiovascular effects of increased blood viscosity.

2 Decreased affinity ('a right shift') — the haemoglobin has a reduced affinity for oxygen and does not take it up freely as the red cell passes through the lungs. Conversely, the oxygen is freely released in the tissues and oxygenation may be normal at much lower haemoglobin levels. As much of the Hb is in reduced form the patients may present with unexplained cyanosis, e.g. Hb Seattle.

M-haemoglobins. Patients with this autosomal dominant condition present in the heterozygous state with cyanosis due to methaemoglobinaemia. These mutant haemoglobins cause the haem iron to be carried obligatorily in the ferric state (Fe^{3+}) and it cannot be chemically or enzymatically reduced. Treatment is unnecessary but other causes for cyanosis should be excluded.

- Cyanotic heart disease.
- Methaemoglobin reductase deficiency.
- Toxic methaemoglobinaemia — nitrates, trinitrin, sulphonamides, nitrobenzene, marking ink.

Defects in haemoglobin synthesis and chain balance

The thalassaemia syndromes

In this complex and diverse group of anaemias there is a reduction in the rate of synthesis of one or more globin chains leading to unbalanced production.

The thalassaemias are named after the specific globin whose synthesis is depressed.

- Most cases are of the α or β type.
- Occasionally two genes may be affected — HbS/β-thalassaemia.
- Some forms produce an abnormal globin chain in addition to the reduction in normal chains — Hb Constant Spring (α variant), Hb Lepore (β variant).

The red cells are deficient in haemoglobin and are hypochromic and microcytic. The excess chains produced by the imbalance (α in β-thalassaemia and β in α-thalassaemia) precipitate into tetramers. These precipitates are removed in the spleen causing cell membrane damage and premature destruction of the cell. In addition, many erythroblasts are destroyed in the marrow causing 'ineffective erythropoiesis'.

Disease expression

Inheritance follows simple Mendelian rules. Children with the severe form of the disease have parents who both usually show minor haematological abnormalities. Thus the terms 'major' and 'minor' were introduced. These clinical descriptions usually correspond to the homozygous and the heterozygous states. Recent work at DNA level and with specific globin synthesis studies has complicated the issue by demonstrating a number of thalassaemia alleles (alternative gene forms). Thus a patient may inherit two different defective genes. These are double heterozygotes rather than homozygotes, and if their clinical picture falls between the major and the minor it is known as 'intermedia'. This is primarily a clinical diagnosis. There are two expressions of β-thalassaemia genes — β^0 with a total failure of β-chain synthesis and β^+ in which synthesis is 3–5% normal.

β-Thalassaemia

This is the best-known and most clinically important form of thalassaemia. It is seen predominantly in Greeks, Italians, and in people from India and South-East Asia.

β-Thalassaemia trait

Prevalence:

- Greeks 10%
- Italians 5–10%
- Indians 1–5%
- SE Asians 5%

The diagnosis is easily made from the haematological picture. The haemoglobin level is low or near normal with a microcytosis (MCV <76 fl), a red cell count over 5×10^{12}/l, and an elevated HbA_2 level (>3%). The HbF level is rarely increased. In addition to hypochromia and microcytosis, target cells are usually present.

Various discriminant functions may distinguish between iron deficiency and β-thalassaemia minor. For example if MCV − [RBC + (Hb × 5) + 3.4] gives a positive result, the diagnosis is likely to be iron deficiency. If negative, thalassaemia is more likely.

These discriminant functions cannot be successfully applied in pregnant women, patients with haematinic deficiency or those who are generally unwell for some reason. Concurrent iron deficiency may mask the diagnosis by reducing haem synthesis and lowering the HbA_2 level, so patients should always be iron-replete before the diagnosis is excluded. β-Thalassaemia trait is usually asymptomatic although the spleen may just be palpable.

4.3 The haemolytic anaemias

β-Thalassaemia major

This is due to homozygous or doubly heterozygous β^0- or β^+-thalassaemia. The condition usually presents in infancy after normal suppression of HbF production with:

- A severe anaemia characterized by microcytosis, target cells, nucleated red cells, and a reticulocytosis.
- Failure to thrive with physical retardation although mental development is normal.
- Jaundice is usually slight.

Hyperplasia of the bone marrow occurs with cortical thinning and abnormal bone structure — 'mongoloid' facies and severe dental malocclusion. There is stunting of growth although the arms and legs are long in comparison to the trunk and there is a decrease in muscle bulk. Without regular transfusions death usually occurs in early childhood. With prolonged survival hepatosplenomegaly occurs, which may be massive with the sequelae of hypersplenism. This results in:

- Shortened red cell survival (autologous and transfused).
- Leucopenia.
- Thrombocytopenia.
- Plasma volume expansion.

The high cardiac output associated with severe anaemia leads to left ventricular hypertrophy and eventually heart failure. As with all the congenital haemolytic anaemias leg ulcers are common. There is increased iron absorption from the gastrointestinal tract in response to the chronic haemolysis and anaemia and this, in conjunction with the repeated blood transfusions, leads to iron overload. Despite a careful transfusion policy death still occurs in the mid to late twenties, principally from the effects of iron overload.

Iron overload:

- Each unit of blood contains 200 mg of iron.
- Normal body stores are approximately 1 g with no active excretion mechanism.

- Tissue damage occurs at about 28 g (age 11–12) when approximately 100 units will have been given.

Three main organ systems are affected:

1 Cardiac — most deaths are ultimately due to heart failure. Acute failure (25%) occurs in those who are more iron-loaded for their age.

Cardiac failure is soon complicated by hepatic, renal and adrenal failure. Hypoxia liberates toxic iron from ferritin.

Chronic recurrent congestive cardiac failure (75%) may persist for some years. Persistent arrhythmias occur. Gross hepatic enlargement is present and there is evidence of multisystem damage.

2 Hepatic — iron deposition leads to fibrosis and ultimately cirrhosis. Liver function tests and clotting studies are abnormal. Extramedullary haemopoiesis may occur and there is a risk of viral hepatitis in the multitransfused.

3 Endocrine — growth failure occurs due to ineffective haemopoiesis in early childhood and later due to endocrine failure. This also causes failure of sexual function so that males are often sterile with no sexual development while females usually have secondary sexual development and menarche with later amenorrhoea.

There are multiple endocrine abnormalities which may progress to produce a symptomatic deficiency due to:

- Reduced insulin secretion — diabetes mellitus.
- Decreased parathormone levels.
- Abnormal thyroid release hormone stimulation with a high TSH.
- Poor adrenal response to ACTH.

Hypoxia may be as important in governing endocrine function as iron overload.

Diagnosis. The classic findings in the blood have been described. Hb electrophoresis must be performed before transfusion. In β^0-thalassaemia no HbA is found, only HbA_2 and HbF. In β^+-thalassaemia some HbA is present, but usually $<15\%$. Globin chain synthesis studies show a marked imbalance. Family studies are always useful in difficult cases.

Management:

1 Blood transfusion. Most centres now adopt a high transfusion policy in an attempt to keep the pre-transfusion Hb level >10 g/dl. This approach should suppress the normal marrow and allow normal growth. It also:

- Reduces the risk of anoxic damage to the endocrine system.
- Reduces enteral iron absorption which may offset the increased load in the blood.
- Prevents hypersplenism.

2 Folate supplements should be given.

3 Iron chelation therapy is necessary. There are no widely available oral agents, and at present the optimum method is desferrioxamine administered as a slow, subcutaneous infusion via a syringe pump. The optimum dose is assessed by measuring iron excretion, and in the average adult is of the order of 2–3 g per day. Vitamin C in moderate doses (200 mg) is often given to aid iron excretion. It does, however, also increase absorption.

4 Splenectomy is indicated if there is significant hypersplenism. This has in the past been necessary at around five years of age. Prophylactic penicillin and pneumococcal vaccine should be given.

Thalassaemia intermedia

This is a clinical condition whose severity lies between the major and minor varieties and does not generally require transfusion. The Hb is between 7 and 10 g/dl.

Causes include:

- Homozygous mild β^+-thalassaemia.
- Homozygous $\delta\beta$-thalassaemia.
- Double heterozygosity for β- and $\delta\beta$-thalassaemia.
- Homozygous β-thalassaemia with hereditary persistence of HbF.
- Homozygous β-thalassaemia with α-thalassaemia.

α-Thalassaemia

Gene mapping has established that there are four α genes, two on each chromosome 16. Four types of thalassaemia are recognized:

- α-Thalassaemia 2 (silent) $(-\alpha/\alpha\alpha)$.
- α-Thalassaemia 1 (trait) $(--/\alpha\alpha, -\alpha/-\alpha)$.
- HbH disease $(--/-\alpha)$.
- Hb Barts hydrops fetalis $(--/--)$.

The silent form of α-thalassaemia and the trait are clinically insignificant except for a mild hypochromia in the latter. There is no simple screening test, and as the α-chain is affected no one type of haemoglobin is abnormal. There are therefore few data on ethnic distribution.

Symptomatic α-thalassaemia is uncommon in Caucasian populations, but α-thalassaemia 2 may occur in up to 25% of blacks. There is a prevalence of 5–10% of carrier status (α-thalassaemia 2 or 1) in the Chinese, and HbH disease and Hb Barts hydrops fetalis syndrome are frequent. Similarly the incidence of carrier status may be as high in Thailand, South East Asia, India, through to Saudi Arabia. The incidence in Greece and Italy is approximately 5%. For definitive diagnosis globin chain synthesis studies are required. The α : non-α ratio is less than 1 in α-thalassaemia.

α-Thalassaemia 2 may be very common in some populations. The MCV and MCH are in the low–normal range. Some Hb Barts (γ_4) may be detectable at birth.

α-Thalassaemia 1 causes a mild anaemia with a MCV which is subnormal. Small amounts of Hb Barts may be detectable at birth. In both these conditions HbA_2, HbF and iron status should be normal.

HbH disease has the clinical severity of β-thalassaemia intermedia, haemoglobin levels of 7–9 g/dl being associated with splenomegaly. The red cells are severely hypochromic and have aggregates of β-chain tetramers (β_4; HbH). At birth up to 25% of the haemoglobin is Hb Barts, which is soon replaced by HbH, which persists at levels around 20%. The haemoglobin may drop precipitously if there is intercurrent infection or pregnancy, and transfusions may be necessary.

Using the supravital stain brilliant cresyl blue HbH shows up as multiple inclusion bodies in the red cell — 'golf-ball' appearance.

Hb Barts hydrops fetalis syndrome (HbBHFs) results from a total absence of α-chain production. Most of the haemoglobin is in tetramers of γ-chains with small amounts of HbH and residual embryonic haemoglobins.

HbBHFs is incompatible with life, usually producing the miscarriage of a non-viable fetus late in pregnancy. The fetus has the appearance of hydrops fetalis with anaemic heart failure. It is important to recognize the carriers with two α-gene deletions so that genetic counselling and antenatal diagnosis can be offered.

Hb Constant Spring is an interesting α-chain variant in which elongation of the α-chain occurs. In South-East Asia many patients with HbH disease lack only two genes, but have inherited the CS gene. When inherited alone the clinical picture mimics α-thalassaemia 2.

δ-Chain thalassaemia

$\delta\beta$-Thalassaemia involves a partial deletion of both δ- and β-chains. It is haematologically similar to β-thalassaemia, but can be distinguished in the heterozygote by a subnormal HbA_2 level and an elevation of HbF up to 15%. The homozygous state is very rare and usually has only HbF.

Hb Lepore mimics β-thalassaemia minor. Most cases occur in Greeks and Italians, and at least three variants have been described. The Lepore chain is a hybrid of the δ- and the β-chains. β-Chain synthesis is reduced, and insufficient Lepore is produced to bind with the α-chain. The A_2 level is normal with a slight increase in HbF with a band of Hb Lepore of about 10%. The homozygous condition resembles a mild form of β-thalassaemia major.

Acquired haemolytic anaemia

Immune-associated

Warm antibody type

Warm autoimmune haemolytic anaemia (AIHA). Red cell destruction occurs due to autoantibodies directed against the patient's own red cells.

- Most are active at 37 °C.
- Autoantibodies can be detected by the direct Coombs (antiglobulin) test (DAGT).

A positive reaction does not always indicate haemolysis and may be found following infection, in renal and connective tissue disorders, and following treatment with certain drugs. Occasionally it may be a chance finding.

Aetiology and clinical features. It is important to determine whether autoimmune haemolysis is primary (idiopathic) or secondary. The main symptom of anaemia provides no clue to aetiology and a detailed drug history is essential. Physical examination may reveal features suggesting a connective tissue disorder or lymphoma. The spleen is usually palpable although massive splenomegaly would suggest an underlying disorder.

In children there may often be a preceding viral infection.

Renal failure is rare except following overwhelming intravascular haemolysis, which is unusual in AIHA.

- In half the patients the condition is idiopathic. Females predominate and AIHA is more common in middle life.
- Haematological malignancies are particularly associated with AIHA, especially chronic lymphatic leukaemia and the non-Hodgkin's lymphomas.

• Autoimmune diseases, particularly the connective tissue disorders such as rheumatoid arthritis and systemic lupus erythematosus, may cause AIHA.
• Many drugs are associated with autoimmune haemolysis, often of unknown aetiology.

Drugs associated with AIHA

1 Drugs that attach to the red cell membrane (hapten).
Penicillin (high-dose, intravenous).
Cephalothin.

2 Immune complex aetiology (innocent bystander).
Quinidine bisulphate.
Chlorpropamide.
Chlorpromazine.
Sulphonamides.

3 SLE-like syndrome.
Hydralazine.
Procainamide.

4 Immune disturbance.
Methyldopa.

Peripheral blood findings. Spherocytes are invariably found in AIHA, although the anaemia is usually macrocytic due to the reticulocytosis. Nucleated red cells are also often found. Leucocytosis occurs transiently during the acute episode, but if this is a lymphocytosis it usually indicates chronic lymphatic leukaemia. Thrombocytopenia is a rare association, and is usually also autoimmune (Evans' syndrome), indicating a poorer prognosis.

Serology. The direct antiglobulin test is positive. The autoantibodies are usually IgG but occasionally may be IgM and IgA. The reaction may give a clue to the aetiology. In SLE the DAGT shows both IgG and complement whereas methyldopa gives a pure IgG reaction. In association with methyldopa the antibody may have rhesus specificity, commonly anti-e. Although 20% of patients taking the drug show a positive DAGT, only 1–2% experience active haemolysis.

Therapy depends on the clinical state and the underlying cause. Any associated disease state should be treated, but the haemolytic process may itself require treatment. If there is a drug association, haemolysis usually ceases within days of stopping the drug although the DAGT may remain positive for months or years.

- Steroids are the mainstay at an initial dose of 1–2 mg/kg/day. Most patients will respond within two weeks, following which slow reduction of the steroids should take place.
- Splenectomy should be considered in steroid failures unless there is a significant contraindication. Between 50 and 75% will respond. *In vivo* counting of radioactivity over liver and spleen after tagging the patient's red cells with ^{51}Cr may be performed and may demonstrate excessive splenic sequestration.
- Immunosuppressive drugs should be considered in steroid/splenectomy failures or when the latter is contraindicated. Azathioprine, cyclophosphamide or chlorambucil are the agents mainly used.
- Blood transfusion may be life-saving in progressively severe anaemia, although it is usually impossible to find totally compatible blood. Despite this, haemolytic transfusion reactions are relatively uncommon.
- Folic acid supplements are needed as stores are rapidly exhausted.
- A variety of other therapies have been tried including thymectomy, antithymocyte globulin, plasma exchange and high-dose intravenous immunoglobulin. None is consistently successful.

Cold antibody type

Cold haemagglutinin disease (CHAD)

Exposure of blood to temperatures less than 37 °C *in vitro* leads to the agglutination of red cells, but whether a fall in temperature is associated with clinical haemolysis depends on the degree of cooling and the thermal range and potency of the antibody. The autoantibodies are usually of IgM type and the incidence is one-quarter of warm AIHA.

Aetiology and clinical features. The condition may be diagnosed unexpectedly by the presence of red cell aggregates on the blood film. More frequently the patient presents with cold-related conditions such as Raynaud's phenomenon or acrocyanosis. An infection may precede the development of cold-related symptoms.

The condition may be idiopathic and often has a slow and insidious onset. It mainly affects the elderly, with an equal sex distribution, and tends to chronicity.

There are a variety of conditions associated with the production of cold antibodies, including:

- Atypical pneumonia (Mycoplasma).
- Infectious mononucleosis.
- Viral infections such as influenza A, mumps, measles and Coxsackie.
- Systemic lupus erythematosus.
- Malignancy such as non-Hodgkin's lymphomas.

Post-infection cold haemolysis tends to produce an acute intravascular haemolytic episode within three weeks of the illness, which is severe while it lasts but subsides spontaneously. In general, CHAD is characterized by a mild chronic haemolysis with haemoglobinuria, haemosiderinuria and a reticulocytosis. The bilirubin is mildly increased. This chronic state is punctuated by acute episodes usually provoked by cold exposure.

Serology. The antibody responsible is IgM and usually has anti-I specificity, although following infectious mononucleosis it is usually anti-i. The thermal amplitude of the antibody varies but tends to be most active at 4 °C and inactive at 37 °C. The wider the range the more severe the condition.

The antibody may be monoclonal or polyclonal depending on aetiology.

- Monoclonal IgM is associated with the lymphoid malignancies and may also be idiopathic.
- In the autoimmune disorders there is usually a mixture of monoclonal and polyclonal immunoglobulin.
- Where haemolysis follows infection the IgM is invariably polyclonal.
- The titres of the antibody tend to be very high in the idiopathic, neoplastic and autoimmune varieties.
- The DAGT may be positive but with complement components alone.
- All blood should be taken with a warm syringe and kept at 37 °C prior to testing. Where possible equipment should be pre-warmed.

Therapy. CHAD is frequently not severe, and the mild chronic haemolysis usually leaves a haemoglobin of 9–12 g/dl. Such patients require no therapy other than avoidance of exposure to cold. Adequate clothing with ear muffs, mittens and wool socks should be worn, and electric-heated gloves are available. Any necessary surgical procedure should be carefully supervised and cooling avoided. Severely affected patients should be given immunosuppressive therapy with chlorambucil or cyclophosphamide. Steroids and splenectomy are seldom of help.

Unfortunately only a minority respond with an increase in haemoglobin and a fall in the cold agglutinin titre and any response is usually slow. In the acute phase plasma exchange may be of benefit.

Blood transfusion can often not be avoided. Compatibility testing must be performed strictly at 37 °C and the blood for transfusion pre-warmed. In general washed cells should be given to reduce the amount of transfused complement, which may exacerbate the haemolysis.

Folic acid supplements should also be given.

Paroxysmal cold haemoglobinuria (PCH)

Aetiology and clinical features. This is a very rare condition which is a sequel to viral (mumps, measles) or syphilitic infections in which a powerful lytic antibody is produced. The main feature is profound intravascular haemolysis following some degree of cold exposure.

- Haemoglobinuria occurs with backache and loin pain.
- Renal failure is a rare concomitant.
- The Donath–Landsteiner test detects the antibody, which is IgG and is directed against the P blood group system.

Therapy. Acute post-infectious forms of PCH terminate spontaneously and only temporary protection from cold is required. In the chronic forms cold protection is more important. Steroid therapy and splenectomy are ineffective. Cells lacking the P blood group are rare, so that if transfusion is required cells should be rigorously prewarmed to 37 °C.

Haemolytic disease of the newborn (HDN) is considered in Section 4.9.

Non-immune associated haemolytic anaemia

Red cells may be prematurely destroyed through increased mechanical stress, acquired defects of the red cell membrane, infections or chemical agents.

Haemolysis caused by red cell trauma

Cardiac haemolysis. Abnormal turbulence set up by diseased or artificial valves can produce variable degrees of haemolysis by direct trauma. It may also occur after Teflon-patch repair of septal defects. Haemolysis is more common if both mitral and aortic valves have been replaced and is particularly associated with the Starr–Edwards valve.

- These patients develop haemoglobinuria and haemosiderinuria, the latter often being sufficient to cause iron-deficiency anaemia.
- The blood film shows marked fragmentation of the red cells with polychromasia.

- Haptoglobins are low.
- Disseminated intravascular coagulation and bacterial endocarditis must be excluded.

March haemoglobinuria. This is a condition characterized by attacks of haemoglobinuria following bouts of strenuous exercise, particularly running on hard surfaces with poor cushioning of the feet. It is said that the red cells rupture in the vessels in the soles of the feet. A similar mechanism may also account for haemolysis following karate blows.

Burns may be associated with haemolysis by direct destruction of the red cells.

Microangiopathic haemolytic anaemia (MAHA). This term encompasses a group of disorders characterized by intravascular haemolysis and red cell fragmentation associated with small vessel disease.

The pathological basis may be an arteritis or fibrinoid necrosis, although disseminated intravascular coagulation itself may produce a microangiopathy. The red cells become fragmented as they pass through the fibrin meshes of small thrombi.

Haemolytic uraemic syndrome (HUS). This term describes the association of acute haemolytic anaemia and renal failure usually in early childhood. There is also:

- Fever.
- Purpura.
- Respiratory distress.
- Drowsiness often leading to coma.

Aetiology is obscure but at least in some cases immune complex-mediated renal capillary damage may occur with local and occasionally disseminated intravascular coagulation. It is likely that an infection is the precipitating event.

- The peripheral blood shows fragmentation and distortion of the red cells with small spherocytes and polychromasia, leucocytosis and thrombocytopenia.
- Blood urea is raised with haematuria and proteinuria.
- The clotting screen is usually normal although fibrin degradation products may be increased.

A variety of treatments have been tried including steroids, heparin, aspirin, dipyridamole, fresh frozen plasma and plasma exchange, but mortality remains high and renal support has a high priority.

Thrombotic thrombocytopenic purpura (TTP). TTP is a disorder of young adults characterized by:

- Severe MAHA.
- Thrombocytopenia.
- Generalized purpura.
- Renal disease.
- Neurological disturbance, including paralysis, coma, and psychiatric problems.

The condition may be acute and rapidly fatal or chronic and relapsing. It may be associated with pregnancy or the connective tissue disorders such as SLE, PAN or rheumatoid arthritis. Treatment options are similar to those tried in HUS although fresh frozen plasma either alone or as part of a plasma exchange appears to be particularly effective.

MAHA is also seen in a variety of other settings:

- Disseminated mucus-secreting carcinoma, especially of the stomach.
- Toxaemia of pregnancy.
- Septicaemia.
- Malignant hypertension.
- Cavernous haemangioma.
- Connective tissue disorders.

Haemolysis related to drug ingestion

A variety of drugs and chemicals may be potential haemolytic agents. Several different mechanisms are involved, both immune and non-immune.

Drug-induced immune haemolysis occurs as a result of at least three different mechanisms (p. 169).

- Hapten formation.
- Innocent bystander mechanism.
- True autoantibody formation.

Red cells are also susceptible to haemolysis by oxidative drugs, especially if there is co-existing G6PD deficiency.

Oxidizing agents lead to denaturation of the haemoglobin with Heinz body formation.

- Normal red cells — dapsone.
- Unstable haemoglobin (Hb Köln) — sulphonamides.
- G6PD deficiency — primaquine, nitrofurantoin, phenacetin, sulphonamides.

Many chemicals if ingested in high enough concentrations will destroy normal red cells.

- Lead (also affects Hb synthesis and causes basophilic stippling).
- Copper.
- Sodium or potassium chlorate causes Heinz body anaemia.
- Arsine gas (a by-product of metal refining).

In addition several physical agents can produce haemolysis.

- 100% oxygen.
- Water if given intravenously.
- Insect stings — bees and spiders.
- Snake venom.

Haemolysis resulting from infection

Haemolytic anaemia following infection may be due to a number of causes.

- Disseminated intravascular coagulation occurs with Gram-negative and Gram-positive infections.
- Bacterial toxins may directly damage the red cell. *Clostridium*

welchii produces a lecithinase which acts on red cell lipoproteins.

- Invasion of red cells by micro-organisms — malaria, oroya fever due to *Bartonella bacilliformis.*
- Haemolytic anaemia may complicate viral infections such as glandular fever and cytomegalovirus infection.

Acquired red cell membrane defects

Liver disease. Red cell survival is shortened in infectious hepatitis, cirrhosis and biliary obstruction. Clinically this is inapparent except in association with other complications.

- Zieve's syndrome occurs in alcoholics with liver disease following a bout of hard drinking.
- Spur cell syndrome is associated with severe hepatocellular disease when markedly deformed red cells are found.

Renal failure. A mild haemolysis occurs with the presence of burr cells in the blood film due to a membrane defect.

Vitamin E deficiency may be associated with haemolysis in the newborn infant. Vitamin E is an antioxidant and its absence allows peroxidation of the membrane lipids. It does not occur in adults.

Paroxysmal nocturnal haemoglobinuria (PNH). PNH is a rare disorder occurring in the third to fifth decades, commoner in women and characterized by chronic intravascular haemolysis with exacerbations associated with haemoglobinuria and a marked thrombotic tendency.

An abnormal clone of haemopoietic stem cells produces abnormal red cells, white cells and platelets. The red cell membrane is sensitive to complement lysis at an acid pH. The cells are also sensitive to low ionic strength solutions such as sucrose.

- The abnormal clone may arise *de novo* or in a previously damaged marrow.
- Chronic haemolysis may occur without haemoglobinuria.

- Classically haemoglobinuria occurs related to sleep.
- Iron deficiency occurs due to haemosiderin loss.
- Venous and arterial thromboses occur. Episodes of unexplained abdominal pain occur, possibly related to thromboses.
- Hepatic vein thrombosis (Budd–Chiari syndrome) may cause portal hypertension and hepatic failure.
- The condition may be superimposed on an aplastic or hypoplastic marrow.
- Low pH-sensitive cell lines occur in the myeloproliferative disorders.

PNH can be diagnosed by finding intravascular haemolysis associated with a positive acid lysis — Ham's test. The sucrose lysis test is also very sensitive.

The disorder is chronic with a survival of many years. Death is usually due to recurrent thromboses, particularly intra-abdominal, although the development of acute leukaemia is described. A variable neutropenia and thrombocytopenia are seen. Treatment consists of general support.

- Transfusion with washed red cells if anaemia is severe.
- Iron supplementation although this may exacerbate the haemolysis.
- Anticoagulation if thrombosis occurs.
- Androgens, steroids and splenectomy have all been tried with little benefit.

Pregnancy is hazardous and seems to be associated with an increased incidence of thrombosis. The contraceptive pill is contraindicated in patients with PNH.

4.4 Non-malignant white cell disorders (acquired)

White cells can be classified into two types depending on the presence of granules, although both arise from the same pluripotential stem cell (Section 3.4).

4.4 Non-malignant white cell disorders (acquired)

• Granulocytes	Multiple lobes • neutrophils • eosinophils • basophils Lobulated • monocytes	myeloid series
• Non-granulocytes	• lymphocytes • plasma cells	lymphoid series

A variety of regulatory mechanisms have been postulated based on *in vitro* culture studies.

- Colony-stimulating factor (CSF) or colony-stimulating activity (CSA).
- Neutrophil-releasing factor (NRF).
- Prostaglandin E — inhibits colony growth of the committed myeloid progenitor cell (CFU-GM).
- Lactoferrin — inhibits CSA production.

The normal values of white cells in the blood vary with age (*see* Table 3.2). The total count tends to be higher in childhood due to a higher lymphocyte count. Neutrophils are present in adult numbers after the first year of life and total adult levels of all cells are reached by 18 years.

Leucocytosis

Leucocytosis is commonly the result of an infection, but more rarely may be a feature of the anaemia of chronic disease. It describes an increase in leucocytes above the normal range and in intense infection counts may persistently remain at quite high levels ($>25 \times 10^9/l$).

Neutrophil leucocytosis

Neutrophil leucocytosis is arbitrarily defined as a neutrophil count greater than $7.5 \times 10^9/l$. Causes include:

4.4 Non-malignant white cell disorders (acquired)

Physiological. Exercise, emotion, pregnancy, and labour.

Pathological (acute inflammatory response):

- Infections — bacterial (not a feature in typhoid or paratyphoid). Not seen in most common viral infections.
- Tissue destruction — trauma, burns, post-operative, subarachnoid haemorrhage, coronary thrombosis, hepatic necrosis.
- Metabolic — diabetic ketoacidosis, gout, Cushing's disease.
- Malignant disease — disseminated or necrotic tumours (especially with liver deposits).
- Acute blood loss and haemolysis.

Leukaemoid reactions occur when the stimulus is intense and are particularly described in disseminated tuberculosis and disseminated malignancy. The condition is so called because it mimics chronic granulocytic leukaemia (CGL) haematologically. Distinguishing features include:

- The peripheral blood shows an increase mainly in mature neutrophils. Occasional 'band' forms and metamyelocytes are present but myeloblasts are unusual.
- Toxic granulation is present.
- The leucocyte alkaline phosphatase score is high in the reactive state but very low in CGL.
- CGL usually has the presence of the marker Philadelphia chromosome.
- The spleen is rarely enlarged in the leukaemoid reaction.

Eosinophil leucocytosis

Eosinophil leucocytosis is present when the eosinophil count is greater than 0.4×10^9/l. Their function is uncertain but they increase moderately in a wide variety of conditions and may be involved in protection of the body surface against foreign protein.

- Allergy, especially asthma, hay fever and urticaria.
- Parasitic infections, particularly when there is tissue or blood-

stream invasion. Parasites especially associated with eosinophilia are roundworm (Ascaris), hookworm (Ancylostoma), Toxocara, and tapeworm (Taenia). In endemic areas there may be a persistent eosinophilia.

- Eczematous states.
- Drug reactions — penicillin, sulphonamides, chlorpromazine.
- Aspergillus infections.
- Connective tissue disorders — especially polyarteritis nodosa.
- Malignant disorders — Hodgkin's disease, metastatic carcinoma.
- Eosinophilic leukaemia and CGL.
- Gastrointestinal disorders — inflammatory bowel disease.
- Tuberculosis and other conditions causing granuloma formation.

The hypereosinophilic syndrome is a condition in which the cause of the eosinophilia cannot be identified and there is profound general disturbance with weight loss, fever, rashes, splenomegaly and pulmonary or cardiac disorders. The features merge with Loeffler's syndrome of pulmonary eosinophilia and Loeffler's endocarditis. When the proportion of immature forms increases in the blood or bone marrow, and if a chromosomal abnormality is identified, the diagnosis of eosinophilic leukaemia must be considered.

Basophil leucocytosis

Basophil leucocytosis is considered when the absolute count is greater than 0.1×10^9/l. This may be seen in urticaria pigmentosa, mastocytosis and myxoedema, but a marked and persistent increase is usually related to the myeloproliferative disorders.

- In CGL an increasing basophil count is a serious prognostic sign and usually heralds blast transformation.

Monocytosis

Monocytosis occurs when the count is greater than 0.8×10^9/l. The monocyte is part of the acute inflammatory response and is the circulating form of the tissue macrophage. Monocytes predominate in chronic inflammatory lesions.

- Bacterial infections — tuberculosis, brucellosis, typhoid and paratyphoid, bacterial endocarditis.
- Protozoal infections — malaria, kala-azar.
- Virus infections — infectious mononucleosis; although many of the atypical cells are lymphocytes.
- Carcinoma.
- Ulcerative colitis and Crohn's disease.

In malignant conditions there is a spectrum of disease affecting the macrophage/monocyte system and classification depends on whether the disorder is localized or more generalized. The following conditions are described:

- Histiocytosis X.
- Histocytic medullary reticulosis.
- True histiocytic lymphoma.
- Acute monoblastic leukaemia.

Lymphocytosis

Lymphocytosis is the term used to describe an increase of lymphocytes above the normal range. This range varies with age, being highest at birth and falling to adult levels by the mid-teens. The level may be increased 'absolutely' or 'relatively' in comparison to the neutrophil counts, and it is therefore important to look at the total number as well as the percentage in the peripheral blood.

Lymphocytosis occurs readily in children as a response to almost any infective challenge and is often persistent. Prolonged lymphocytosis in adults however almost invariably has a neoplastic basis. Important causes include:

- Viral infections, especially glandular fever and cytomegalovirus.
- Any infection in children, especially whooping cough.
- Tuberculosis and brucellosis.
- Typhoid and paratyphoid fevers.
- Toxoplasmosis and mycoplasma pneumonia.
- Secondary and tertiary syphilis.

- Autoimmune thyroid disorders.
- Carcinoma.
- Lymphoid neoplasms.

Infectious mononucleosis (glandular fever, IM)
This is the commonest cause of membranous tonsillitis or persistent sore throat and may cause pronounced haematological changes giving rise to some diagnostic difficulty.

- The incidence is about 2–6/10 000 of the population per year, and the 15–20 age group is most affected.
- The incubation period lies between four and eight weeks.

Aetiology. Infection is caused by the herpes virus known as the Epstein–Barr virus (EBV). Infectivity is low and the agent is transmitted in saliva.

- Most infections are acquired in early childhood and pass unrecognized.
- Primary infection acquired in late adolescence is accompanied by the clinical disease.
- EBV is found in Burkitt's lymphoma in Africa and nasopharyngeal carcinoma in the Far East, with high EBV antibody titres.

Clinical features. Typically the lymph nodes in the neck are generally enlarged, there is a sore throat and a fever may persist for 1–2 weeks.

- The throat shows clusters of fine haemorrhages on the hard and soft palate with a white exudate on the tonsils. When severe, inflammatory oedema may impair swallowing or breathing.
- Lymph node swelling may persist for up to one year.
- The spleen is palpable in 50%.
- Liver enzymes are abnormal in up to 90% but overt jaundice only occurs in 5–10%.
- A few patients show evidence of myocarditis, nephritis and pancreatitis.

- The chest X-ray may show pulmonary infiltration.
- A maculopapular rash develops during the second week, usually on extensor surfaces. The rash may be precipitated by ampicillin.
- Periorbital oedema is uncommon but well described.
- Nervous system involvement occurs in about 1% and ranges from meningitis and encephalitis to neuritis. Recovery is complete but may be delayed.

Peripheral blood features:

- The total white cell count is normal during the first week and occasionally a leucopenia is found.
- A moderate lymphocytosis develops during the second week and may reach 30–40 × 10^9/l.
- The cells are large and morphologically abnormal with dense basophilic, vacuolated cytoplasm, a lobulated or indented nucleus and scalloped edges where they abut an adjoining cell.
- They have the phenotype of T-suppressor lymphocytes.
- They are also found in the other conditions which mimic IM and are thought to be the body's response to the infection of B-cells by the infecting organism.
- The atypical cells may be seen for several months.
- There may be a false-positive Wasserman reaction and the rheumatoid factor and ANF become transiently positive.
- Cold agglutinins may appear (anti-i specificity) and produce a haemolytic anaemia and occasional immune thrombocytopenia is seen.

Diagnosis is confirmed by a positive screening test for horse or sheep cell agglutinins in the patient's blood (known as heterophil antibodies).

The classic Paul–Bunnell test measures serial dilutions of serum before and after adsorption by guinea-pig kidney cells and ox cells. The antibody is adsorbed by the ox but not by the guinea-pig cells. Other heterophil antibodies are present in 'normal' sera but are adsorbed by the guinea-pig cells. If the test is negative despite clinical suspicion a diagnosis of CMV or toxoplasmosis should be considered. The heterophil antibody is present in high titres during the acute illness and may be detected for up to eight months.

Treatment. Despite the alarming appearances of the throat, secondary bacterial infection is rare and antibiotics should be avoided. Treatment is symptomatic and bed rest is advisable until the temperature settles.

Steroids should be used for respiratory obstruction, and in view of the hepatitis the patient should be advised to abstain from alcohol.

Persistent fatigue and inability to concentrate are common complaints but complete recovery can be assured.

Angioimmunoblastic lymphadenopathy

• This is a non-neoplastic proliferation of unknown cause. There is a marked lymphoid activation with a polyclonal hypergammaglobulinaemia and frequently a Coombs-positive haemolytic anaemia.

This has previously been considered to be a B-cell proliferation, but is now increasingly associated with T-cell tumours. Systemic symptoms of the type associated with Hodgkin's disease are found and there is generalized lymphadenopathy and hepatosplenomegaly. Skin rashes are common. Diagnosis is made by lymph node biopsy, prognosis is poor and malignant transformation often occurs.

Leucopenia

Depression of the total white cell count below the accepted normal level of 4×10^9/l defines leucopenia. The term usually implies a reduction in neutrophils or lymphocytes in the blood since although the other cell lines may be reduced their total numbers are such that they do not affect the absolute white count.

A reduction in the white cell count makes the patient particularly at risk from infection, especially once the neutrophil count falls below 1.0×10^9/l. The reduction in neutrophils reduces the ability of the body to localize and limit infection so that systemic spread is rapid and commensals that live on the body surface are a particular risk.

Neutropenia

Moderate reductions may be picked up by chance, but once the count falls below 0.5×10^9/l the patient invariably develops infection. Vulnerable sites include:

- Throat.
- Chest.
- Perianal area.

Causes include:

• Bone marrow damage	Ionizing radiation
	Cytotoxic drugs
	Drugs and chemicals
	Severe infection
	  tuberculosis
	  septicaemia
	  infectious hepatitis

• Bone marrow obliteration	Neoplasia
	  acute leukaemia
	  lymphoma
	  myeloma
	  metastatic carcinoma
	Osteosclerosis

• Immune damage	Drugs
	  chlorpromazine
	  sulphonamides
	Infections
	  glandular fever
	  Mycoplasma
	Systemic lupus erythematosus
	Isoimmune
	  neonatal
	  post-transfusion

- Hypersplenism — Felty's syndrome
- Deficiency states — Vitamin B_{12}, Folic acid
- Paroxysmal nocturnal haemoglobinuria
- Aplastic anaemia

Drug causes of bone marrow failure are particularly important. A number of agents cause direct marrow suppression, e.g. cytotoxic agents, DXT. Others affect the marrow much more variably, either as a dose-related effect or idiosyncratically. The list is long, and no exhaustive collection can be given. It is therefore important to consider this mechanism in all patients with any evidence of marrow failure (*see* p. 138).

Lymphopenia

When the absolute lymphocyte count falls below 1.5×10^9/l there may be associated increased susceptibility to bacterial and viral infections, particularly if both humoral and cell-mediated arms are affected. Causes include:

- Hodgkin's disease.
- DXT and cytotoxic agents.
- Anti-lymphocyte globulin administration.
- Steroid administration and Cushing's syndrome.
- AIDS.
- Uraemia.
- Systemic lupus erythematous.
- Kwashiorkor.
- Intestinal loss in intestinal lymphangiectasis and Whipple's disease.
- Sarcoidosis.

Acute illness is often associated with a transient lymphopenia and is generally due to a mixture of increased destruction and reduced production.

4.5 Acute leukaemia

Classification is based on the predominant cell type and is divided into two main types:

- Acute myeloblastic leukaemia (AML).
- Acute lymphoblastic leukaemia (ALL).

These are often further subdivided depending on morphological, immunological and enzymatic characteristics of the cells.

- The incidence of AML is approximately 2.4/100 000 in the western world.
- The incidence of ALL is 1–2/100 000.
- 4% of all cancer deaths are due to leukaemia.
- The ratio of deaths from acute and chronic leukaemia is 1.8 : 1.0.
- Nearly 50% of patients with ALL, but only 5% with AML, are less than 15 years old.
- There is a rapid increase in incidence of AML in the over-50 age group.

Aetiology

Ionizing radiation

- Survivors of atomic bomb explosions have a 10- to 15-fold increase in the incidence of leukaemia compared with control populations.
- Practising radiologists had an increased incidence before the potential dangers were recognized.
- Therapeutic irradiation for non-malignant disease such as ankylosing spondylitis and to induce artificial menopause is also associated with an increased risk of leukaemia.

Viruses

Gene mapping has identified specific areas in the genome of cells where changes produce a proliferative advantage without differentiation. The relationship between viruses and these specific areas may lead to identification of the cause of leukaemia and possible lines of treatment.

RNA tumour viruses induce a variety of tumours in experimental animals, but the evidence in man is more tenuous. The genomes of these viruses may carry transformation-specific genes (oncogenes) coding for part or all of a protein required for the initiation and maintenance of the transformed phenotype. Some viruses may act by inducing the expression of oncongenes in the host cells. Evidence for their involvement has been demonstrated by finding:

- Reverse transcriptase, a DNA polymerase, in some leukaemic cells.
- Virus-like particles have been demonstrated in some cases of AML.
- Nucleotide sequences in the DNA of leukaemic cells are found which are similar to those found in some animal leukaemia viruses.
- Following bone marrow transplantation relapse may occur in donor cells.
- The type-C retroviruses, which include the human T-lymphoma leukaemia viruses (HTLV), have been implicated in a variety of tumours including Sezary syndrome and mycosis fungoides.
- The Epstein–Barr virus (EBV), a DNA virus, is strongly related to two malignancies, Burkitt's lymphoma and nasopharyngeal carcinoma.

Chemicals

Toxic environmental chemicals and some therapeutic agents are known to be leukaemogenic. Two types are particularly strongly associated:

- Benzene, toluene and other petroleum derivatives.
- Alkylating agents, in particular melphalan, cyclophosphamide and chlorambucil. Most patients develop AML, often with a hypoproliferative preleukaemic phase. There may be a latent period of 3–12 years.

Hereditary factors

• Host susceptibility affects the development of leukaemia in certain disorders and probably plays a role in the outcome of most cases of leukaemia.

• Acute leukaemia occurs with great frequency in Down's syndrome — trisomy 21 — and in two autosomal recessive disorders associated with chromosomal breakage — Bloom's syndrome and Fanconi's anaemia.

Acquired haematological disorders and other diseases

Leukaemia has been described in association with a variety of malignant and non-malignant conditions. In each case it must be considered whether the two are unrelated, the leukaemia is part of the natural evolution of the disease or has been induced by therapy.

• There is a clear association between AML and Hodgkin's disease, non-Hodgkin's lymphoma, multiple myeloma, breast cancer and ovarian cancer.

Pathogenesis

The principal cell found in acute leukaemia is the 'blast', which is the earliest recognizable cell in any particular cell line. It is likely that the leukaemic stem cell is altered in some way so that normal differentiation of the progeny does not occur. Development is arrested in acute leukaemia at the level of the blast so that there is a gradual accumulation of these long-lived immature cells. These primitive cells gradually replace the normal marrow elements leading to a peripheral pancytopenia. As the numbers increase they gradually spill out into the peripheral blood providing the typical appearances at presentation.

Diagnosis

The diagnosis of acute leukaemia can only be made by examination of peripheral blood and bone marrow films stained with Romanowsky dyes. The basis of diagnosis is cell morphology often aided by cytochemical staining characteristics. The use of immunological techniques to detect antigens and other cell surface molecules is particularly valuable in differentiating lymphoblasts.

Electron microscopy, often in conjunction with cytochemistry, may be valuable.

Cytogenetic abnormalities are present in many of the leukaemias. In some they are clonal and have diagnostic and prognostic significance (*see* Section 3.13).

Acute myeloblastic leukaemia (AML)

AML involves the myeloid series of the bone marrow and is the

Table 4.7 Differentiation of leukaemic blast cells.

	Lymphoblast	Myeloblast
Nucleoli	Usually one	More than two
Cytoplasm	Scanty High nuclear/cytoplasmic ratio	Abundant Low nuclear/cytoplasmic ratio
Auer rods	Absent	Present
Sudan black	Negative	Posititve
PAS	Strong block positive	Negative or weak background positive
Acid phosphatase	Negative except in T-lymphoblasts	Positive
Naphthol AS acetate esterase	Negative	Positive — myeloid resistant to fluoride; monocytic abolished by fluoride
Chloracetate esterase	Negative	Positive

most common type of leukaemia in adults. There is an equal sex incidence, and below the age of 50 a steady incidence of disease. Over the age of 50 the incidence increases rapidly, mainly in men.

Clinical features

The major features result from bone marrow failure and the onset is usually acute.

- Anaemia causes pallor, palpitations and dyspnoea. Occasionally in the older patient angina pectoris may develop.
- Neutropenia causes infection, which may begin locally, often in the gut, chest or skin, but rapidly becomes systemic.
- Thrombocytopenia causes bleeding, often with petechiae and purpura in the skin, but intracranial haemorrhage is an important cause of death.
- Infiltration of the gums, skin and perineum is seen in monocytic types.
- A combination of infection, haemorrhage and infiltration in the mouth or the anus may result in serious, painful and distressing lesions.

Classification (French–American–British – FAB)

Category	*Characteristics*
M0	Undifferentiated
M1	AML without maturation
M2	AML with 10–20% of cells differentiating
M3	Acute promyelocytic leukaemia (APML)
M4	Acute myelomonoblastic leukaemia (AMML)
M5	Acute monoblastic leukaemia
M6	Erythroleukaemia
M7	Megakaryoblastic leukaemia

Eighty per cent of newly diagnosed AML falls into the categories of M1, M2 and M4, with a predominance of M2.

Promyelocytic leukaemia (APML)

APML occurs in 7% of cases and is predominantly in the younger age group. It is associated with a high incidence of disseminated intravascular coagulation (DIC) and severe haemorrhagic phenomena. This is due to the procoagulant activity of the granular cytoplasmic fraction.

If the patient survives the early phase of treatment, his survival is better than average with 20% surviving five years. The majority have the chromosomal abnormality t(15q+;17q−).

Monocytic leukaemia

There are two forms:

1 Associated with myeloid differentiation,

2 A pure monoblastic proliferation.

Controversy exists as to whether these are distinct entities or are part of a continuing spectrum. The M5 variety (monoblastic) is associated with a high WBC and tissue infiltration, in particular gum hypertrophy, skin infiltrates and lymphadenopathy. Splenomegaly is also frequently found.

The serum and urinary lysozyme levels are raised and may be responsible for renal tubular dysfunction which is seen in this group, leading to hypokalaemia.

Response to cytotoxic treatment is poor and patients are more prone to CNS infiltration.

Acute erythroleukaemia

The erythroid element of the marrow exceeds 30% and the erythroblasts are abnormal with lobulation of the nucleus, multiple nuclei, nuclear fragments and megaloblastoid changes. Myeloblasts are often also increased and Auer rods are often present. The PAS stain is usually positive and the iron stain may show ring sideroblasts.

Acute megakaryoblastic leukaemia

A rare and fulminant form of AML. This condition usually presents with a severe pancytopenia without organ enlargement. Bone marrow aspiration is usually unsuccessful due to increased marrow fibrosis. Megakaryoblasts show abnormal differentiation and can be identified by platelet myeloperoxidase, antiplatelet monoclonal antibodies and characteristic electron microscope appearances.

Clinical management of AML

Survival in patients with AML has improved markedly over the last 20 years. In the early 1960s a temporary return of normal bone marrow function occurred in less than 10% of patients following cytotoxic therapy, with recurrence and death usually within one year. By the mid-1980s up to 75% were achieving a complete remission with a 50% survival rate of 24 months and up to 10–15% achieving cure.

However, the majority of patients with AML still die of the disease. The difficulty in treating AML results from a number of points.

- The older age group of patients.
- The drugs used are not selective against the leukaemic cells.
- To achieve remission it is a prerequisite to induce profound bone marrow hypoplasia.

The increase in CR rate and improvement in length of remission is mainly due to the development of progressively more myelosuppressive antileukaemic therapy. The achievement of these benefits has required parallel improvement in the management of infection and haemorrhage.

Prognostic features associated with poor survival

- Age greater than 60 years.
- AML as a secondary disease or with documented preleukaemic phase.
- Abnormal chromosomal karyotype.
- A high WBC and thrombocytopenia at presentation.
- Serious infection at diagnosis.

Treatment aims to reduce the number of leukaemic cells from the presentation load of 1×10^{12} to less than 1×10^{9}. At this stage it is unusual to detect any leukaemic cells in the blood or bone marrow, which look essentially normal. This state is called complete remission.

This early treatment with its inevitable period of bone marrow aplasia requires expert support by experienced staff in a properly equipped environment with a full range of back-up services. In general, particularly for the younger patient, treatment should be confined to the larger centres.

Support care

Psychological. The patient and his family need a detailed discussion, tailored to the individual, about the disease, the treatment plan and side-effects of treatment, with an emphasis that the aim of treatment is to return to normal life. Many conflicting emotions arise during the treatment, including anger, resentment and fear, and it is important that the patient has a member of staff who will be available to discuss and explain these feelings. A number of interviews with the patient and relatives are essential for psychological support to be effective.

Physical:

- Reverse barrier nursing is important in the early phase of treatment to protect the patient from the outside environment.
- Equipment, foodstuffs, and clothing should be sterilized.
- When the patient is handled gowns and gloves should be worn and meticulous handwashing is essential, but masks are of doubtful value and place an additional barrier between patient and attendant.
- Oral non-absorbable antibiotics are used to reduce endogenous infection from the gastrointestinal tract,
- Microbiological screening from mouth, skin, stool and urine should be performed.
- Right atrial tunnelled catheters are now used routinely in most centres.

At the onset of treatment a thorough assessment of cardiac, renal, hepatic and respiratory function should be made.

Red cell transfusions

- The haemoglobin concentration should be maintained above 8 g/dl.
- Plasma-reduced blood is usually given to prevent reactions, but filtered or washed cells may be necessary for some multitransfused patients.

Platelet transfusions

Thrombocytopenia is universal following ablative therapy, and prior to ready access to platelet concentrates haemorrhage was a major factor in the death of 70% of patients.

Petechiae are rare if the platelets are greater than 30×10^9/l, life-threatening haemorrhage occurring when the count is less than 20×10^9/l, although the rate of fall and concurrent infection are important.

The patient should be examined daily for haemorrhagic manifestations, particular attention being paid to:

- Fundi.
- Urine microscopy for red cells.

Platelet supplements are usually given as concentrates obtained fresh from random donor blood processed at blood transfusion centres.

- One unit of platelet concentrate from 475 ml of blood contains $0.5–1.0 \times 10^{11}$ platelets.
- 30% are lost during processing and 30% do not circulate, being sequestered in the spleen.
- It is usual to give up to six pooled bags daily ($3–4 \times 10^{11}$ platelets).
- Supplements are given daily until bleeding ceases or the bone marrow recovers.
- Requirements are greater if there is DIC or intercurrent infection.

- If resistance occurs HLA-matched platelets obtained by a cell separator may be required.

Infections

All patients become neutropenic during therapy, and the majority will develop a fever. If fever develops suitable specimens for culture and sensitivity should be taken and a broad-spectrum combination of antibiotics started. The combination will depend on previous experience within the unit or the patient's own previous surveillance cultures. Infections now account for between 25 and 50% of deaths in adult leukaemia.

- Positive cultures occur in 40–60% of cases.
- Lack of neutrophils reduces the local reaction so that any infection rapidly becomes systemic.
- Local signs of infection, e.g. pus, are unusual.
- Multiple infections occur in up to 20% of cases.
- Opportunistic infections occur that are rarely seen in normal practice (especially Candida and Pneumocystis).
- Blood products or the disease itself may cause pyrexia.

Bacterial infections are most common during the neutropenic phase. Untreated they are rapidly fatal.

Gram-negative infections have always predominated, but with the greater use of long-term indwelling catheters Gram-positive infections are now seen in up to 30% of cases. However, the Gram-negative infections tend to be more rapidly fatal, and treatment is designed to cover these in the first instance.

In a large study by the European Organisation for Research and Treatment in Cancer four bacterial species accounted for 65% of all pathogens isolated.

- *Escherichia coli*.
- *Staphylococcus aureus*.
- Klebsiella spp.
- *Pseudomonas aeruginosa*.

While *Staphylococcus aureus* was the second most frequently identified cause of infection (16%), the Gram-negative group comprised 61% of all isolated organisms.

- Pneumonia is the most common serious infection, mostly caused by Gram-negative rods, especially *Pseudomonas aeruginosa*.
- The increasing use of indwelling intra-atrial catheters has been accompanied by an increase in infection by the 'skin organisms'; coagulase-negative staphylococci (mainly *Staphylococcus epidermidis*), the coryneforms and the viridans streptococci.

In most units empirical treatment consists of an aminoglycoside in conjunction with an antipseudomonal ureidopenicillin. Changes are made depending on the response, culture data and the patient's clinical state.

Fungal infections. The majority of patients undergoing treatment for AML develop mucositis. This is primarily due to the drugs used but is invariably complicated by candidal overgrowth, Candida being a usual mouth commensal. The non-absorbable antibiotic regimens contain antifungal agents such as nystatin or amphotericin lozenges or elixir. In the severely immunosuppressed patient, particularly following prolonged neutropenia, systemic candidiasis may develop, and intravenous amphotericin should always be considered in a pyrexial patient who is not responding to broad-spectrum antibiotics.

Viral infections. With intensive immunosuppressive therapy the incidence of herpetic infections is increasing, now affecting up to 50% of patients. The infection may be localized as a cold sore or mucositis but can disseminate involving brain, lungs or other tissues. Morbidity and mortality were high until the advent of acyclovir, a specific antiviral agent. It is available as a topical agent but should always be given parenterally in the immunosuppressed patient.

Cytomegalovirus infection may also occur but is only important in the bone marrow transplant group where mortality is high. In AML it usually causes an unexplained fever that slowly resolves.

Specific antileukaemic therapy

Treatment strategy in AML:

1 Remission induction.
2 Consolidation.
3 (a) Allogeneic BMT.
  (b) Autologous BMT.
  (c) Maintenance therapy — drugs used earlier + other agents.
    — ? immunotherapy.
4 Craniospinal prophylaxis.
5 Late intensification.
6 Stop treatment.

The aim of specific antileukaemic therapy is to return the bone marrow to a state of normality. As the drugs used have an equivalent cytotoxic effect on nomal and leukaemic cells, it is usual to produce a hypoplastic marrow during initial therapy. Failure to achieve a complete remission (CR) may be due to primary failure of the chemotherapy or failure to maintain the patient through the cytopenic phase. The most effective drugs at present are the anthracyclines (adriamycin, daunorubicin), cytarabine and thioguanine. Most regimens involve these in combination giving 1–3 doses of the anthracycline, with daily administration of the other two agents up to a total of 10 days.

The aim has been to intensify the initial regimen with improved leukaemic cell kill leading to a greater chance of achieving CR. There is no convincing evidence that any one regimen is superior to the others, CR rates lying between 70 and 80%. With optimum supporting care resistant leukaemia still accounts for up to 10% of early deaths. Individual differences in reported series reflect the patient population, support care and experience, rather than inherent differences in the treatment.

- The achievement of remission is the important initial aim.
- Failure to achieve CR is associated with very poor survival.
- Once CR is achieved the aim is to prevent recurrence.

- If no further treatment is given following achievement of CR then relapse is almost inevitable.

It has, therefore, been customary to follow remission induction treatment with consolidation therapy and some form of maintenance treatment.

It seems increasingly likely that prolonged remission and cure are associated with very intensive early treatment and some form of consolidation. The value of maintenance treatment is marginal and may be counterproductive when it comes to treating relapse. Using these principles:

- Up to one-fifth entering CR will not relapse.
- Median duration of first CR may approach three years.
- Attempts to prolong CR using immunotherapy have met with only marginal success.
- Bone marrow transplantation attempts to cure the disease by giving very intensive chemoradiotherapy followed by allogeneic or autologous bone marrow rescue (*see later*).

CNS prophylaxis. CNS leukaemia is becoming increasingly recognized with prolonged survival in AML. It is particularly common in monoblastic leukaemia and those who present with very high blast counts. The incidence is approximately 10%, lower than in ALL. Prophylaxis using intrathecal treatment with or without cranial irradiation should be considered, particularly in the younger patients.

Treatment in relapse. Once relapse has occurred there is no possibility of cure, although further brief CR may be achieved. Each patient who enters CR should be evaluated for allogeneic bone marrow transplantation, and if not suitable consideration should be given to harvesting and storing autologous marrow. This is increasingly used in CR to intensify treatment but can be given in relapse. Allogeneic BMT in relapse gives poor results, and an attempt should be made to achieve a second CR before using this technique.

4.5 Acute leukaemia

Acute lymphoblastic leukaemia (ALL)

This commonest malignant disease of childhood with a peak incidence between the ages of four and five accounts for 20% of all leukaemias. There is a slight excess of males to females. Almost 85% of childhood leukaemia is ALL; the incidence falls in adolescence then rises steadily throughout life.

Clinical features

The condition is clinically indistinguishable from AML, presenting often with symptoms and signs of bone marrow failure. The history is usually short and there is no preleukaemic phase.

- The WBC may be normal but an absolute neutropenia is usual.
- Blasts can be identified in the peripheral blood.
- Bone and joint pains are frequent associations, and an initial diagnosis of juvenile rheumatoid arthritis is not uncommon.
- Lymphocytosis is a common reaction to infection in childhood, and care must be taken to exclude infectious mononucleosis, pertussis and rubella.
- Physical signs may be absent but lymphadenopathy with or without hepatosplenomegaly is often seen.
- A mediastinal mass is seen in T-cell ALL, often with a very high WBC.

Classification

This can be done on morphological criteria, but ALL is now more commonly subdivided by immunological surface membrane characteristics using monoclonal antibodies and certain enzyme estimations.

Morphology:

Category	*Characteristics*
L1	Small, monomorphic
L2	Large, convoluted and heterogeneous
L3	Burkitt-cell type

Membrane markers:

Table 4.8 Classification of childhood ALL.

	B/T markers	Anti-ALL serum	Tdt	Ia	Morphology	Incidence
Common ALL	Neg	Pos	Pos	Pos	L1	70%
Null ALL	Neg	Neg	Pos	Pos	L1	9%
T-ALL	T	Neg	Pos	Neg	L1 or L2	20%
B-ALL	B	Neg	Neg	Pos	L3	1%

ALL can be subdivided into four subgroups using a panel of markers.

- T-cell markers — spontaneous rosettes with sheep RBC (E-rosettes).
  — anti T-cell serum both monoclonal and polyclonal heterologous thymocyte antisera.
- B-cell markers — surface (Sm Ig) and cytoplasmic (C Ig) immunoglobulin. Monoclonal antisera can demonstrate monoclonality of the cell line.
- Anti-common ALL antisera detect an antigen (c ALL) on B- and T-cell precursors.
- Terminal deoxynucleotidyltransferase (Tdt) detected chemically or by immunofluorescence is present in common null and T-ALL but rarely in B-ALL or AML.
- Anti Ia-like serum detects the HLA–Dr complex and is found on normal myeloid and B-lymphocyte but not T-lymphocyte progenitors.

Using these, and other, markers it is possible to differentiate most types of ALL.

- Common ALL is the type seen in most children with ALL. The blasts are small with inconspicuous nucleoli and little cytoplasm. They fall into the L1 category. They do not have characteristics of T- or B-cells but are probably of pre-B cell lineage.
- Null ALL is more common in adults. The cells lack the common ALL antigen but have high levels of Tdt. The cell type tends to be L1.

Survival is poorer than in common ALL.

• T-cell ALL is predominantly a disease of males and is associated with a mediastinal mass and high blast count. It responds initially to treatment but CR is short. The blasts are of early T-cell lineage and may be L1 or L2 morphological type.

• B-cell ALL is rare. The blasts resemble those in Burkitt's lymphoma and have surface immunoglobulin. The cells are classically L3. Survival is poor and the cells are usually refractory to treatment. CNS leukaemia is very common.

Adult ALL

The incidence of common ALL is half that in children. The majority have L2 morphology and up to 20% present with a positive Philadelphia chromosome, without evidence of previous CML. The outlook is much worse than in childhood ALL.

Clinical management of ALL

Treatment in 'standard' risk ALL can be summarized in four main phases.

Treatment strategy in ALL:

1 Remission induction — vincristine.
— prednisolone.

2 Consolidation.

3 CNS prophylaxis — cranial DXT.
— intrathecal methotrexate.

4 Maintenance (2–2$\frac{1}{2}$ years) — mercaptopurine.
— methotrexate.

5 Stop treatment.

Remission can usually be achieved in 4–6 weeks in over 90% of children. Standard treatment incorporates oral prednisolone and intravenous vincristine; it is relatively non-myelotoxic and can be given to some extent on an outpatient basis. Anthracyclines can be added and may increase the CR rate but do increase the risk of early complications and are not necessary in all cases. Once CR is achieved an intensification of the treatment is given as consolidation. This utilizes drugs such as L′-asparaginase and VP16 (epipodophylotoxin).

Without craniospinal prophylaxis meningeal leukaemia will develop in over half of children while in haematological remission. It is conventional to use cranial irradiation and intrathecal methotrexate.

Maintenance chemotherapy is given using at least two drugs continued for 2–3 years. This phase of treatment can be given as an outpatient with visits every 3–4 weeks for blood testing.

When to stop therapy

There is no evidence that continuing treatment for longer than 2–3 years increases long-term remission and may increase morbidity. If treatment stops at 2.5 years, up to 20% will relapse in the next 12 months, but survival then reaches a plateau. Thus up to 75–80% of those in remission for the first 2.5 years may be cured.

- Survival is worse in boys, partly due to testicular relapse, the testis being a sanctuary site. Unless specific testicular prophylaxis has been given, bilateral testicular biopsies should be carried out at the end of the maintenance period.
- CNS leukaemia will develop in up to 10% despite craniospinal prophylaxis.

Prognostic features

- A high WBC is a poor prognostic feature irrespective of cell type.
- Boys do less well than girls.
- T- and B-cell markers indicate poorer survival.
- Age is an important variable with survival better between three and seven years.
- CNS leukaemia at presentation is a poor feature.
- Rapid achievement of CR is associated with a good outlook.

It may be possible to tailor treatment depending on the expected response, saving a number of children from unnecessarily aggressive treatment.

Support care

General bone marrow support may be necessary at presentation, but as the usual regimens are less intensive than in AML this is not usually prolonged.

Psychological support for patients' parents and other relatives is particularly important, especially when dealing with children. This must not be overlooked if treatment is carried out as an outpatient, as the parents may feel unable to express themselves if they have not developed a close relationship with one or more of the hospital staff.

Complications of treatment

In ALL the antileukaemic treatment differs from that in AML but is not altogether free from side-effects.

The treatment is immunosuppressive without severe myelosuppression and, as profound neutropenia is rare, the risks of bacterial infection are reduced. Non-bacterial infections are a more severe hazard and they account for 5–10% of deaths in remission, being the main reason to avoid 'over-treating' good prognostic cases. Most are due to viral infections.

• Varicella zoster can cause disseminated infection, pneumonia and encephalitis.

• Measles may cause giant cell pneumonia and encephalitis even without the rash.

Contact with these infections should be avoided, and if it occurs immune globulin should be given. Varicella zoster responds to acyclovir.

• These children should never receive any live vaccine.

Infection with the protozoon *Pneumocystis carinii* is a serious complication causing pneumonitis, but the use of cotrimoxazole has reduced its incidence and severity.

CNS prophylaxis may cause:

- A transient syndrome of somnolence, ataxia and lethargy occurring six weeks post treatment.
- A subtle impairment of intellectual development, in particular mathematical ability.
- A severe demyelinating leucoencephalopathy with progressive deterioration, dementia, ataxia and coma. This is fortunately rare.

Growth and development tend to be normal. Fertility is variable, tending to be normal in girls.

Treatment in relapse

A second remission may be achieved in up to 80%; this is easier if relapse has occurred off treatment. The second CR tends to be short-lived. At this stage bone marrow transplantation should be considered although there remains a significant risk of leukaemic recurrence.

Bone marrow transplantation (BMT) for leukaemia

The main objective of BMT is the cure of the underlying haematological malignancy without the need to undergo prolonged chemotherapy. With the exception of childhood acute lymphoblastic leukaemia, a cure cannot be expected with conventional chemotherapy.

The principle of BMT is that the use of bone marrow rescue allows the doses of chemotherapy and/or radiation to be increased to such a level that the patient's leukaemic cell burden will be eliminated. It is usually given so that autologous bone marrow reconstitution is unlikely, and the associated immunosuppression also reduces the likelihood of graft rejection.

Who to transplant

In *acute lymphoblastic leukaemia* the majority of children are cured by combination chemotherapy (70%). Certain poor prognostic groups should be considered for BMT in first remission. These

include patients with:
- B-cell ALL.
- High blast counts (>100 × 10^9/l) in T-cell or common ALL.
- Chromosomal karyotype abnormalities.
- And those over the age of 14 and under 45.

In *acute myeloblastic leukaemia* long-term survival will only be seen in 10–20% and all suitable patients should be considered for BMT in first remission.

Chronic myeloid leukaemia cannot be cured by conventional treatment. Results from BMT are encouraging in the first chronic phase and all suitable patients should be evaluated. Results in the accelerated phase are less good and those in acute transformation very poor.

Choice of donor
Most transplants are performed betweeen sibling pairs (allogeneic transplantation) who are identical for the major histocompatibility system.
- In the UK about 30% of patients with acute leukaemia have an available donor.
- In order to expand the donor pool use is now being made of haplotype-identical related pairs and HLA-matched unrelated pairs.

Immunosuppression and conditioning
Most preparative regimens for allogeneic BMT comprise total body irradiation in association with cytotoxic drugs. Irradiation is given either as a single dose or fractionated at a dose rate of 2–20 cGy per minute up to a total dose of 1200 cGy. Most transplant teams use high-dose cyclophosphamide (60 mg/kg on two days) as additional cytoreductive and immunosuppressive therapy. It is conventional to use mesna with the cyclophosphamide to bind the acrolein metabolite which causes urothelial toxicity with haemorrhagic cystitis. In aplastic anaemia the TBI is usually unnecessary. Other agents and

approaches are currently under evaluation, such as busulphan, cytarabine, antilymphocyte globulin and total nodal irradiation.

Bone marrow harvest

Donor marrow is collected under general or spinal anaesthesia by multiple punctures from the posterior and anterior iliac crests and sternum. At least $2–3 \times 10^8$ nucleated cells per kilogram recipient weight are collected. In an adult this represents 700–1000 ml of total volume. This may be infused intravenously into the recipient unmanipulated, although many centres now undertake depletion of immunocompetent T-lymphocytes from the donor marrow in an attempt to prevent graft versus host disease. The putative pluripotential stem cell will recirculate and seed the recipient bone marrow space. Neutrophils usually appear soon after day 10, platelets and red cells developing more slowly. ABO incompatibility is not a contraindication to allografting. The donor marrow should be depleted of red cells prior to infusion, and if the recipient has a high isoagglutinin titre this may be reduced by plasma exchange. Erythopoietic recovery may be delayed by several weeks.

Outcome of bone marrow transplantation

1 Successful engraftment.
2 Graft failure.
3 Leukaemic relapse.
4 Death from lethal complications of the procedure:
 (a) Infection.
 (b) GVHD.
 (c) Pneumonitis.

Support care

The major cause of early death is infection. The majority are due to reactivation or invasion by organisms carried by the host. Support care follows the same guidelines used in the treatment of acute leukaemia. Since the regimens are more toxic and myeloablative, greater care is necessary. The degree of mucositis is generally greater; limiting oral food intake and parenteral nutrition should be considered.

Other measures include:

- Consideration of prophylactic acyclovir and cotrimoxazole to prevent herpes simplex and Pneumocystis infection.
- The donation of CMV-negative blood products and/or hyperimmune CMV serum.
- All blood products should be irradiated.

Graft failure

A relatively rare occurrence in early series, graft failure is now reported in up to 30% of cases in some series undergoing BMT using T-depleted bone marrow. It is probable that the depletion technique removes important stroma and support cells that are necessary for graft viability.

Leukaemic relapse

This occurs frequently when BMT is undertaken in relapse, second CR or in blast transformation of CML, but in early series occurred in less than 10% of allogeneic grafts. The incidence of relapse in syngeneic grafts in first-remission AML has been reported to be as high as 50%, and it has been suggested that GVHD has an antileukaemic effect. It is likely that the incidence of recurrent leukaemia will be higher following T-depleted BMT due to loss of this graft versus leukaemia effect.

Graft versus host disease (GVHD)

GVHD is due to minor histocompatibility antigen differences in the recipient recognized by donor T-lymphocytes. Up to 70% may develop some form of acute GVHD. This is manifest by fever, skin rash, diarrhoea and liver dysfunction in varying combinations. Moderate disease may respond to steroids, but if it progresses it is generally unresponsive and may be fatal in 30–40%. There have been numerous approaches in prevention, and manipulation of donor marrow to remove T-cells has reduced the incidence to approximately 10%.

Acute GVHD may progress to chronic GVHD. This causes varying degrees of liver dysfunction, often in association with a debilitating scleroderma-like collagen vascular disease. This occurs in 10–25% of patients who are particularly susceptible to Gram-positive and opportunist infections because of their disordered immune system. The severe form of GVHD is often complicated by cytomegalovirus infection and interstitial pneumonitis, which is usually fatal. Patients with chronic GVHD may respond to azathioprine.

Approaches to prevention of GVHD:

1 HLA identity and MLC non-reactivity between donor and recipient.

2 Treatment of recipient after BMT — methotrexate.
— cyclosporin A.

3 Removal of T-lymphocytes from donor marrow:
Monoclonal antibodies against T-cells.
Physical methods — soy bean lectin.
— sheep red cell rosetting.
— centrifugation.

Interstitial pneumonitis

This type of pneumonitis is a frequent complication of allogeneic BMT, occurring in up to 60%. The patient has a dry cough, dyspnoea and a diffuse interstitial pulmonary infiltrate. More than half the cases are due to CMV, and the mortality rate in this group may reach 90%. Pneumonitis may also be due to *Pneumocystis carinii*, and viruses other than CMV are implicated, e.g. adenovirus. Radiation injury to the lung is an exacerbating factor, and previous exposure to fibrogenic drugs such as busulphan may increase the incidence.

Results

AML in first remission. Disease-free survivals of up to 60% have been reported, although a more realistic figure at three years is probably 40%. Long-term disease-free survival in second or later CR is substantially lower.

ALL. In poor-risk ALL four-year disease-free survival is of the order of 60% with a risk of relapse of nearly 30%. Standard-risk ALL should be treated with conventional chemotherapy and transplantation undertaken in second CR, although BMT at this stage has a lower chance of producing long-term survival and there is a higher chance of relapse.

CML. BMT in the first chronic phase is associated with disease-free survival of 75% at two years. In the accelerated phase survival is less good at 35%; in blast transformation survival is very poor at less than 10%. A small number of patients transplanted in first chronic phase have had a cytogenetic (Ph′ positive) relapse but the clinical tempo of the disease is then apparently extremely slow.

Autologous marrow transplantation

Transplant-related toxicity increases with the age of the recipient, and many patients are therefore excluded from allografting. For this group and for those without a donor the use of autografting is being considered.

The concept of achieving CR and then collecting and cryopreserving marrow cells, for use in the management of relapse, is not new. This concept is being extended to treatment in remission and for certain solid tumours. Greater numbers of patients can be treated and the problems of graft rejection and GVHD are not present. Two problems need to be considered:

- The suitable regimen of chemoradiotherapy to prepare the patient.

- Whether the harvested marrow needs treatment to remove or inactivate residual leukaemic cells — 'purging'.

Preliminary results show the procedure to be safe, and studies in acute myeloblastic leukaemia autografted in first remission show disease-free survival of up to 30% over two years, giving results which are not significantly different from allografting.

Pre-leukaemia and myelodysplastic syndromes

These categories cover an increasingly recognized population with varying degrees of pancytopenia who do not have overt leukaemia. They tend to occur in the older age groups and the history may stretch over months or years.

As with AML and ALL there has been an attempt at classification by the French–American–British Co-operative Group.

- Refractory anaemia without excess blasts.
- Refractory anaemia with ring sideroblasts (RARS).
- Refractory anaemia with excess blasts (5–20%) (RAEB).
- Refractory anaemia in transformation (blasts 20–30%) (RAEBT).
- Chronic myelomonocytic leukaemia (CMML).

Presentation may be incidental or may be due to symptoms of a cytopenia.

- Anaemia is usual often with a marked macrocytosis and the HbF level is occasionally raised.
- Neutrophils are often reduced in number and are often hypogranular with Pelger–Huet forms.
- The NAP score is low or normal.
- Platelets show giant forms.
- Monocytes are often increased and may be the only abnormal feature of the peripheral blood.
- The bone marrow is hypercellular in all categories.
- Erythropoiesis is megaloblastic with multinuclearity.
- Granulopoiesis is left-shifted with or without an increase in blasts.
- Megakaryocytes often display micronuclearity.
- Chromosomal abnormalities are relatively common.

Virtually all overt leukaemia is AML, but this does not always occur. Not surprisingly those with excess blasts develop AML more frequently and more rapidly, this condition occurring in up to 40% with RAEB and CMML.

Treatment is not usually offered during the dyshaemopoietic phase, often due to patient age. However, once leukaemia has occurred, survival is poor, rarely exceeding three months, with little response to specific therapy. Culture studies may help predict survival. Those with a normal growth pattern tend to do better with a slower development of bone marrow failure or overt leukaemia.

4.6 Myeloproliferative disorders

Classification of the myeloproliferative disorders is difficult because of the way in which:

- There is a spectrum of disease without clearly defined boundaries.
- One disorder is capable of transforming into another.

Properly the term should be confined to:

- Clonal stem cell defects in which one or more elements of the peripheral blood are present in excess without a complete failure of maturation.

When considering this subject, it is also necessary to discuss other causes of increased peripheral blood cell numbers, erythrocytosis being particularly important.

Traditionally, acute leukaemia is excluded from the discussion except when it arises as consequence of one of the accepted myeloproliferative disorders.

Polycythaemia rubra vera (PRV)

This is a disease of adults. Clinical features due to the increase in cell numbers are:

- Plethora.
- Headache.
- Tinnitus.
- Visual disturbance.

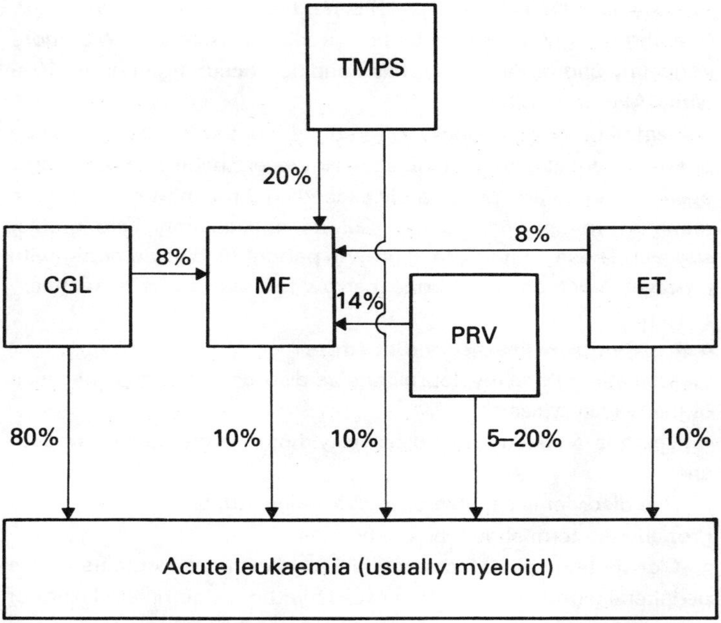

Key: TMPS = transitional myeloproliferative syndrome
CGL = chronic granulocytic leukaemia
MF = myelofibrosis
PV = polycythaemia rubra vera
ET = essential thrombocythaemia

Fig. 4.3 The myeloproliferative disorders and their transitions. Percentage figures represent approximate incidence of transition in direction shown.

- Thrombosis and peripheral vascular occlusion.
- Gout.

In addition, many patients complain of:

- Pruritus made worse by contact with hot water, and
- The spleen is often palpable. In the later stages of the disease it may be massively enlarged.

Associated problems are:

- Peptic ulceration.
- Hypertension.

The main features in the peripheral blood are an elevated Hb, PCV, and RBC count (*see* p. 46) and blood viscosity. The white cell count and platelet count are often increased, the latter sometimes arising above 1000 $\times$ 10^9/l. The film is usually normal morphologically, although there may be a slight left shift in the granulocyte series, and large platelets may be visible. There is often an increase in:

- Neutrophil alkaline phosphatase (NAP).
- Uric acid.

In the absence of any complicating factors there is no need to examine the bone marrow, which is hypercellular. The red cell mass should be measured but will be elevated in most types of polycythaemia and is not of differential diagnostic value.

Differential diagnosis

Secondary polycythaemia is due to:

- Altitude.
- Cyanotic heart disease.
- Hypoxic lung disease.
- Erythropoietin production in:

1 Kidneys — tumour or obstruction.

2 Liver — hepatoma.

3 Pelvis — uterine fibroids.

4 Nervous system — cerebellar haemangioma.

- Abnormal haemoglobins having increased oxygen affinity or defective oxygen-carrying power.

If the diagnosis of PRV is obvious, with such specific features as splenic enlargement, leucocytosis, thrombocytosis, hyperuricaemia and raised NAP, the causes of secondary polycythaemia need not be pursued. When there is doubt and no other clinical clues are present, consider:

- A chest X-ray.

- Urine examination.
- Intravenous urography.
- Haemoglobin analysis.
- An oxygen dissociation curve.

Stress polycythaemia

This term refers to patients with an elevated haemoglobin concentration, red cell count and blood viscosity but normal red cell mass and reduced plasma volume. They are often hypertensive. When dehydration and the use of diuretics have been excluded, there remains a group of patients who have an increased risk of thrombosis. In general treatment is not given unless the PCV is greater than 0.54.

Management of PRV

The main aim is to normalize the peripheral blood and suppress myeloproliferation.

1 Simple venesection will reduce the red cell count slowly but will stimulate platelet production. It is possible to remove up to a litre of red cells isovolaemically using a cell separator, and with this technique platelet counts remain stable. The PCV should be maintained below 0.45 whichever method is used.

2 Radiophosphorus (^{32}P) given intravenously at a dose of about 5 mCi will control myeloproliferation but may cause hypoplasia and the effect is delayed for some weeks. ^{32}P probably also increases the likelihood of transformation to myelofibrosis and acute leukaemia. ^{32}P should be avoided if the diagnosis of PRV is not certain but is particularly useful for patients with very high platelet counts.

3 In microvascular occlusion, especially when the platelet count is high, aspirin 50–150 mg daily brings dramatic relief of pain and may improve tissue perfusion.

4 Allopurinol controls the level of uric acid, especially at the time of ^{32}P injection.

5 Pruritus is very difficult to treat and often fails to respond to antihistamines or any other medication.

Management of other causes of polycythaemia

Venesection is of value in 'stress polycythaemia', and this may apply to the other secondary conditions. Occlusive episodes are less common and performance may be improved at lower PCVs. In practice, it is not usually possible to treat all patients with secondary polycythaemia regularly in this way, and it should be remembered that the cause of their polycythaemia may be reversible.

Haematinics in polycythaemia

After venesection many patients become iron-deficient and develop a normal Hb and PCV with an elevated red cell count. Folic acid deficiency is not uncommon because of increased cell turnover. It is probably best to leave iron deficiency untreated unless rigid control over the red cell mass can be guaranteed.

Folic acid deficiency should be treated, and extra venesections should be performed if indicated.

Natural history of PRV

The median survival can be extended from 2 to 13 years by the treatment outlined above. If patients escape thrombotic disease they are liable to develop myelofibrosis and/or acute leukaemia as part of the natural history of the disease, perhaps accelerated by ^{32}P injection or cytotoxic drugs.

Chronic granulocytic leukaemia (CGL)

This condition is also known as chronic myeloid leukaemia (CML). This is a disease of adults, but there is a similar rare childhood condition which will be considered later. Some patients fail to develop symptoms to begin with and incidental diagnosis is not uncommon. Eventually the following features are likely to appear:

- Malaise.
- Night sweats.
- Shortness of breath.
- Visual disturbance.

- Priapism in men.
- Easy bruising and bleeding.
- A feeling of fullness or pain in the left hypochrondrium due to enlargement of the spleen, which may be massive.
- Gout.

The main feature of the peripheral blood is a very high white cell count which may reach 500×10^9/l. The whole spectrum of granulocytes and their precursors is present, mature forms being most numerous and blasts not usually exceeding 5% at presentation. Basophils and eosinophils are absolutely and relatively increased. The haemoglobin concentration is normal or reduced, and platelets are usually normal or increased in numbers. Other important features include:

- The Philadelphia chromosome (Ph′) is an acquired translocation between no. 22 and no. 9 and is almost a specific marker for CGL. The abnormal chromosome is found in the developing myeloid cells of the marrow but is not present in tissue cells.
- A reduced NAP.
- Hyperuricaemia.
- Serum B_{12} and B_{12} binding protein are high as a result of increased production of transcobalamin 1 by the expanded granulocyte mass.

The bone marrow is solidly hypercellular with a gross increase in developing myeloid precursors. There may be some increase in reticulin at presentation. Blast cells are less than 15% in the chronic phase.

Differential diagnosis

The diagnosis is rarely in doubt as the spleen is almost invariably enlarged and the Ph′ chromosome is present in 96% of cases.

In Ph′-negative cases there may be some confusion with other chronic and subacute myeloid leukaemias, but this is of little clinical consequence.

Patients with leukaemoid reactions usually have a high NAP and the spleen is rarely much enlarged.

Natural history

The median survival of three years reported in the 1920s has remained essentially unaltered because of the inevitable development of fatal acute blast transformation. The survival curve is, however, very skewed and occasional patients live for up to 15 years. Transformation may occur abruptly in 15% and is referred to as 'blastic crisis'. Symptoms may develop in a few days and the marrow is replaced by monomorphic primitive blast cells. The majority of patients become increasingly resistant to treatment with features of acute leukaemia superimposed on the chronic phase (accelerated phase). A small percentage become myelofibrotic (8%) and slightly less develop an extramedullary mass as the first marker of transformation. When acute leukaemia eventually develops the majority of cases are myeloid, but up to 20% are lymphoid in cell type. Indications of transformation are:

- Unexplained fever and malaise.
- Bone pain.
- A rapidly enlarging spleen.
- An extramedullary mass.
- Difficulty in controlling the haemoglobin, white cell and platelet count.
- Increasing basophilia.
- The appearance of blasts in the peripheral blood.

At this time there is often a deterioration in the karyotype due to clonal evolution with the appearance of extra Ph′ chromosome(s), trisomy 8 and other abnormalities (*see* p. 108).

Management

It is important to discuss with the patient the nature of the disease, in particular the fact that a number of years of good health may be possible but that alteration in the character of the disease is inevitable. Whatever is eventually advised, the first step is to improve the peripheral blood. This can be done by:

- Leucaphaeresis if a cell separator is available.

Several procedures are necessary to make much impact on the

white cell count but the cells removed can be stored, frozen and preserved for future use.

- Hydroxyurea up to 3 g daily to reduce the white cell count rapidly.
- Allopurinol 300 mg daily to control the uric acid level.

The higher the white cell count, the more urgent is the treatment. If priapism develops it rarely resolves without surgical intervention.

For patients under the age of 40 with a compatible HLA-matched sibling, bone marrow transplantation (*see* p. 206) should be considered in the first chronic phase. The potential advantage of this approach is the cure of an inevitably fatal condition, but transplantation carries its own risks which cannot be ignored in a disease with a time-course often measured in years.

Patients who reject or are unsuitable for transplantation must continue with conventional treatment. Long-term control of the peripheral blood is often easier with busulphan, with or without thioguanine, because these drugs have a greater suppressant effect on the stem cell. Busulphan should be used cautiously as it is carcinogenic and mutagenic and it can cause permanent bone marrow damage, skin pigmentation and pulmonary fibrosis. There is a suggestion that busulphan may accelerate leukaemogenesis. Survival is similar with all agents, but hydroxyurea has the advantage of lack of chronic toxicity and rapid reversibility of inadvertent overdosage. Busulphan is best reserved for persistent thrombocythaemia. α-Interferon is being evaluated in some centres and has been shown to suppress Ph′+ve clones. Whether this improves survival awaits long-term trials.

Once transformation begins the outlook is bleak.

1 The accelerated phase may be controlled by more vigorous conventional chemotherapy.

2 Myelofibrosis often requires support with transfusion, and folic acid deficiency should be treated if it arises.

3 Splenectomy or splenic irradiation is of little value.

4 Frank leukaemia is usually treated with a regimen suitable for the cell type involved but results are often disappointing. Attempts at autologous transplantation using stored buffy coat cells and formal allogeneic transplantation in the acute phase have not generally been successful.

Childhood CGL

This condition should not be regarded as a form of CGL. It usually affects very young children who have:

- Enlargement of lymph nodes, liver and spleen.
- A characteristic skin rash.
- Anaemia, leucocytosis and thrombocytopenia.
- Increased HbF.

The Philadelphia chromosome is not present but other karyotypic abnormalities may be found. The outlook is poor.

Essential thrombocythaemia

As in other myeloproliferative disorders adults are chiefly affected and there is a close relationship with PRV. Paradoxically the clinical features include both:

- Abnormal bleeding from cuts, trauma and surgery.
- A thrombotic tendency, especially microvascular occlusion causing pain and necrosis in the extremities with normal peripheral pulses. Large vessel occlusion also occurs.

The spleen may be enlarged, but this is often not the case as splenic atrophy occurs following repeated infarction. The peripheral blood shows a marked increase in platelet numbers, which often exceed $1000 \times 10^9/l$, and there is great variation in platelet size. Sometimes micromegakaryocytes, which look rather like lymphocytes, may be found in the blood as well. Leucocytosis, polycythaemia or anaemia is common.

Other laboratory findings are:

- Raised NAP.
- Hyperuricaemia.
- Platelet functional defects:
  1 Prolonged bleeding time.
  2 Spontaneous platelet aggregation when platelet-rich plasma is stirred in a curette.

3 A failure of the release reaction in response to adrenaline and collagen.

The bone marrow can be difficult to aspirate and there is a great increase in megakaryocytes, particularly in the paratrabecular areas. Reticulin is often increased and there may be frank myelofibrosis.

Differential diagnosis

The causes of thrombocytosis are given on p. 55. Essential thrombocythaemia may merge into PRV, myelofibrosis and megakaryocytic leukaemia.

Management

1 The main priority is to reduce the platelet count as this will largely correct the bleeding and thrombotic tendency.

Initially:

- Hydroxyurea 1–2 g daily with
- Allopurinol 300 mg daily.

will have a rapid effect, and then:

- ^{32}P will provide long-term control in the older age groups.

2 Symptoms of microvascular occlusion usually respond to aspirin 50–150 mg daily and this does not seem to increase the bleeding tendency. Aspirin can be stopped when the platelet count has been corrected.

3 Any surgical procedure should be avoided if at all possible until medical treatment has taken effect. Vascular surgery or amputation can often be avoided in this way.

4 Folic acid deficiency should be treated if it arises.

Busulphan and other drugs acting mainly on the stem cell should be avoided where possible as prolonged survival without leukaemic transformation often occurs. They may also exacerbate marrow fibrosis. Transitional states should be treated on their merits.

Myelofibrosis

Fibrosis of the bone marrow is a reaction to myeloproliferation rather than a part of the process itself and may occur during the course of any of the disorders already discussed. It is thought to be caused by the release of platelet-derived growth factor from the increased numbers of abnormal megakaryocytes. It can also arise by itself. Patients present with the symptoms of anaemia and splenic enlargement; unexplained fever is sometimes found and haemorrhage is not uncommon.

The peripheral blood is leucoerythroblastic, often with grossly abnormal red cells and normoblasts, an elevated white cell count including precursors, and thrombocytopenia or thrombocytosis. Bone marrow cannot usually be aspirated and trephine biopsy shows increased reticulin with or without other signs of myeloproliferation. Useful investigations are:

- NAP, which is usually raised.
- Uric acid.
- Folic acid, which is very commonly deficient.

Differential diagnosis

Primary myelofibrosis has to be distinguished from that due to:

- Other myeloproliferative diseases.
- Other causes of bone marrow infiltration.

Management

1 The cornerstone of management is blood transfusion support. Many patients develop white cell antibodies, and blood should be filtered, especially if reactions occur. Iron overload is a theoretical complication of treatment but is not usually a practical problem and chelation therapy is not indicated.

2 Folic acid and allopurinol prophylaxis is worthwhile.

3 Myelosuppressive cytotoxic therapy is valuable for thrombocytosis or leucocytosis but rarely makes much impact on spleen size.

4 Splenectomy is worth considering in patients with very large spleens and an increasing transfusion requirement.

A clinical decision is often as good as one based on detailed isotopic investigation. The post-operative period can be very difficult, mainly because of the haemostatic defect. Unfortunately splenic irradiation is not very helpful.

Transitional myeloproliferative states (agnogenic myeloid metaplasia)
Many cases of myeloproliferation cannot be fitted precisely into the four major conditions described above. Up to 10% of patients display features that may be found in all categories without demonstrable chromosome abnormality. The clinical picture often resembles myelofibrosis but the marrow is not fibrotic at presentation and the main feature is myeloid metaplasia. The spleen is usually palpable, there is teardrop poikilocytosis and leucoerythroblastosis. Progress to myelofibrosis may eventually occur followed by blastic transformation, although mean survival is over five years. Chemotherapy may be useful at an early stage to control cellular proliferation.

4.7 Lymphoproliferative disorders

This group of disorders includes all neoplastic proliferation of lymphoid cells. The important group consisting of acute lymphoblastic leukaemia (ALL) has been considered separately as it produces unique clinical features. It requires a distinctive therapeutic approach and is more closely related to the other haemopoietic precursor malignancies (Section 4.5).

The lymphoproliferative disorders are, in general, diseases of mature lymphocytes affecting both B- and T-cell types, but include the immunoglobulin-secreting plasma cells. Hodgkin's disease is usually considered with this group because of similar clinical features. There is increasing evidence, however, that it is a separate entity.

Approximately 90% of non-Hodgkin's lymphoma is of B-cell lineage; the remainder is of T-cell origin. Cell markers are available which reflect biological differences between the various cell types and the various stages of maturation which are not readily identified by conventional cytology and morphology. Membrane and enzyme markers may also be used, as in the acute leukaemias. These may be relatively simple, e.g. surface and/or intracytoplasmic immunoglobulin, or require sophisticated analysis of the DNA for immunoglobulin gene rearrangements, or the T-cell receptor genes. It is generally felt that the malignancies reflect the characteristics of the cell type at the level that maturation arrest occurs (*see* Section 3.4). The association between disease characteristics, cell type and stage of maturation is particularly established in the B-cell tumours, as shown in Fig. 4.4, but less so in those affecting T-cells. There are two major groups of T-cell leukaemia/lymphoma. The first in which blast cells predominate, have an immature phenotype (thymic or pre-thymic) and predominate in children and young adults. They include T-ALL and T-lymphoblastic lymphoma. The second group are morphologically and immunologically mature and have a post-thymic phenotype. These are rare, affecting almost exclusively adults, and include T-CLL, T-PLL, adult T-cell lymphoma/leukaemia and the cutaneous T-cell lymphomas.

Table 4.9 Lymphoproliferative disorders (excluding Hodgkin's disease and ALL).

B-types	Lymphocytic (B-CLL) Prolymphocytic (B-PLL) Hairy cell (HCL)
	Non-Hodgkin's lymphomas (NHL)
	Plasma cell dyscrasia multiple myeloma (MM) benign monclonal gammopathy heavy chain disease amyloidosis Waldenstrom's macroglobulinaemia (WM)
T-types	Lymphocytic (T-CLL) Prolymphocytic (T-PLL) Adult T-lymphoma/leukaemia (ATLL) Sezary syndrome

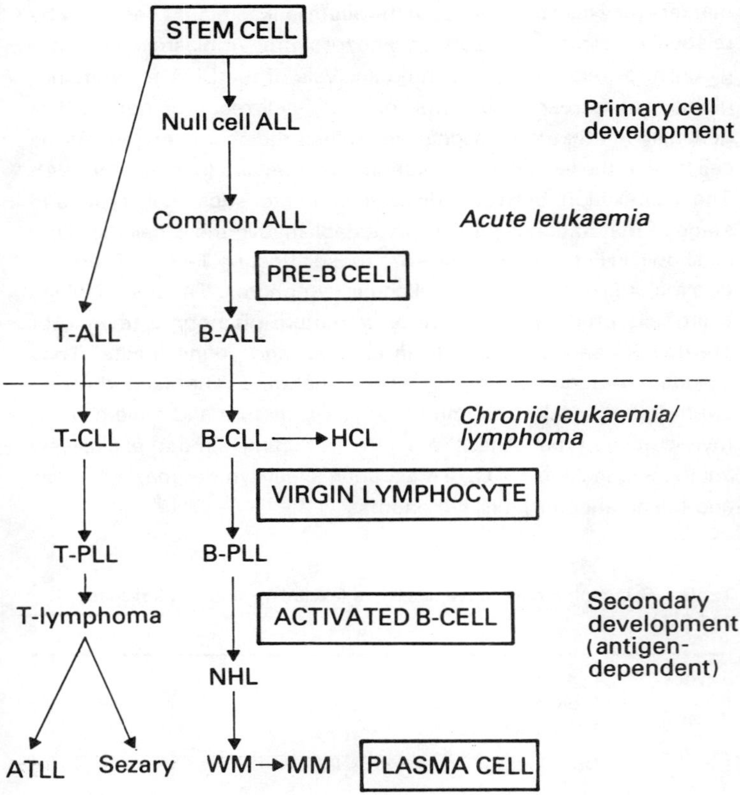

Fig. 4.4 Lymphoproliferative disorders and their relationship to cell maturation.

Chronic lymphocytic leukaemia

This is the commonest form of leukaemia in the West. The incidence is 3 per 100 000, constituting 25% of all leukaemic cases. The mean age of onset is 60 and it is nearly twice as common in men. The cause is unknown but there is an increased familial incidence.

- 98% of cases have a B-cell phenotype; 2% are T-cell.

- The cells are uniform, small, mature-appearing lymphocytes.
- Isotyping shows that the heavy chains on the surface and in cytoplasmic immunoglobulin are generally restricted to IgM or IgM + IgD. The surface imunoglobulin is weakly staining.
- Monoclonality is implied by finding either kappa or lambda light chains in any one case.
- The B-cells form rosettes when mixed with mouse erythrocytes. The rosetting is enhanced by pretreatment of the lymphocytes with neuraminidase.
- The lymphocytes are immunologically incompetent.
- The T-cells in B-CLL are abnormal in both number and function.

The clonal nature of the B-lymphocytes allows a diagnosis to be made even when there is a mild lymphocytosis.

Clinical features

For most patients the disease is indolent, and in 25% the diagnosis is an incidental finding. Presentation is typically with symptoms of anaemia or following discovery of enlarged lymph nodes.

Physical examination is often completely negative. However, as the disease progresses lymphadenopathy, enlargement of the liver and spleen and finally signs of marrow failure occur. This is used as a means of clinical staging.

Table 4.10 Rai's staging classification for chronic lymphocytic leukaemia.

Stage 0	Absolute lymphocytosis ($>15 \times 10^9$/l)
Stage I	Absolute lymphocytosis plus enlarged lymph nodes
Stage II	Absolute lymphocytosis plus enlarged liver and/or spleen (lymphadenopathy need not be present).
Stage III	Absolute lymphocytosis plus anaemia (<10 g/dl) (secondary causes for anaemia should be excluded; physical signs need not be present.)
Stage IV	Absolute lymphocytosis plus thrombocytopenia ($<100 \times 10^9$/l) (exclude immune thrombocytopenia; physical signs need not be present)

Laboratory findings

The peripheral blood should have a lymphocyte count $>15 \times 10^9$/l. Lower counts can be accepted if the immunological characteristics are typical. Counts greater than 250×10^9/l are not unusual and a high white count alone causes few symptoms. A film of the blood shows numerous 'smudge' cells. Anaemia when present is normochromic and normocytic.

- Up to 10% have a positive direct antiglobulin test although not all of these develop frank haemolysis.
- Thrombocytopenia is usually due to marrow failure although occasionally immune thrombocytopenia occurs.
- Hypogammaglobulinaemia occurs in 50% involving all three immunoglobulin classes.

The combination of B- and T-cell defects leads to a variety of infections.

- Pneumococcal pneumonias.
- *Mycobacterium tuberculosis*.
- Viral infections, e.g. herpes simplex and zoster.
- Candidal infections.

The bone marrow is usually diffusely infiltrated, as are lymph nodes and spleen.

Clinical course

The disease shows a very variable progression. The clinical staging implies a steady increase in lymphocytic infiltration affecting bone marrow, lymph nodes, spleen and liver, and finally extensive marrow infiltration. There is much individual variation. The disease may remain static for many years, or even regress, but in general there is steady progression. Mean survival is greater that five years. This varies from 12 years in stage 0 to less than a year in stage IV.

Transformation of B-CLL

True malignant transformation of B-CLL is uncommon but two major forms are described.

1 'Prolymphocytoid' with an increase in prolymphocytes. The

WBC progressively rises with enlarging tumour mass. Response to therapy is poor.

2 'Immunoblastic', which may take the form of a lymphomatous change (Richter's syndrome) or a blast crisis resembling acute leukaemia.

Treatment

The disease is incurable but its diagnosis does not necessitate specific therapy. Stage 0–II should be observed and treatment only given if there is progression or if there is troublesome or unsightly lymphadenopathy. If bone marrow failure occurs, therapy should be given. Chlorambucil as single-agent therapy is often effective. In non-responders combination therapy using cyclophosphamide, vincristine and prednisolone is worth trying.

Corticosteroids are effective in temporarily reducing tumour mass but increase the risk of infection and are usually reserved for autoimmune haemolytic anaemia.

Radiotherapy is used for localized tumour mass, and fractionated total body irradiation may have a role in end-stage disease. Immunoglobulin replacement therapy has been tried in recurrent infections but its value is uncertain.

T-cell chronic lymphocytic leukaemia

Less than 2% of patients with CLL have a proliferation of T-cells. The cells usually show the phenotype of cytotoxic/suppressor cells. Morphologically the cells are large with numerous azurophilic granules and correspond to the large granular lymphocytes. Splenomegaly is usually present but skin infiltration and lymphadenopathy are rare.

The lymphocyte count is only moderately increased ($<30 \times 10^9$/l) with proportional marrow infiltration. It is usual to find some degree of peripheral blood cytopenia, with neutropenia the most common, followed by thrombocytopenia and red cell hypoplasia.

- Splenectomy is often performed to correct the neutropenia in view of the splenomegaly and mild marrow infiltration. This rarely corrects the defect and often leads to an increased lymphocyte count.

• A surprising number of these patients also suffer from rheumatoid arthritis and may be misdiagnosed as Felty's syndrome.

Treatment is rarely indicated, but if required low-dose chlorambucil is usually effective.

Prolymphocytic leukaemia

This variant of CLL is a distinct clinicopathological entity. The typical cell is about twice the size of the small lymphocyte. It has a large prominent nucleolus, well-condensed nuclear chromatin and a moderate amount of cytoplasm.

• 80% of the cases are due to B-cell proliferation and the rest are of T-cell origin.

• The B-cells have denser surface immunoglobulin than the cells in B-CLL and do not form mouse red cell rosettes.

• The T-cells have both helper and suppressor phenotypes on the cell surface. Clinically the disease presents with a very high WBC (T > B), splenomegaly tends to be massive and lymphadenopathy is unusual.

Skin infiltration may be seen in T-PLL.

Response to conventional chemotherapy is usually poor.

Splenectomy may relieve symptoms and slow progression of the disease. However, survival tends to be short.

Hairy cell leukaemia (HCL)

This disorder mainly affects males in the fifth and sixth decades.

• Characteristic hairy cells form a variable proportion of the nucleated cells in the peripheral blood.

• In most cases the cells demonstrate B-cell characteristics. They have variable rosette formation with sheep red cells, which may be enhanced by phytohaemagglutinin stimulation, and synthesize and secrete immunoglobulin.

Clinically, HCL is characterized by pancytopenia and splenomegaly without lymphadenopathy. Presentation is usually with non-specific symptoms but infection, haemorrhage or splenic pain may occur. There is a marked neutropenia and monocytopenia which increases the infection risk. The incidence of tuberculosis is particularly high.

Laboratory features

Tha bone marrow is difficult to aspirate and trephine biopsy is usually necessary to make the diagnosis. There is a diffuse infiltration of hairy cells and an increase in reticulin. The hairy cells have fine surface projections which are best seen by phase contrast microscopy. The tartrate-resistant acid phosphatase reaction is positive in most cases.

Electron microscopy demonstrates a ribosome–lamellar complex in the cytoplasm in 50% of cases.

Course

The disease is slowly progressive with a mean survival of five years. Chemotherapy rarely affects the progression and may increase the infection risk.

Splenectomy often relieves the pancytopenia and the majority benefit to some degree.

α-Interferon has been shown to be effective in reversing the pancytopenia and may reduce the need for splenectomy.

Solid tumours of the lymphoid system

Conventionally these tumours are divided into two main subtypes.

- Hodgkin's disease (HD).
- Non-Hodgkin's lymphoma (NHL).

Although there are superficial similarities between the two groups, especially in presentation and clinical features, they are in fact relatively distinct. Hodgkin's disease has a characteristic histological pattern, and advances made in staging and treatment have particularly affected management; this has not been the case in NHL. This latter group is much more heterogeneous with considerable differences in disease behaviour, varying from indolent to very aggressive. In children NHL often mimics acute lymphoblastic leukaemia.

Hodgkin's disease

This condition is characterized by the presence of the Reed–Sternberg giant cell — a binucleate cell — and its mononuclear counterparts. It generally arises in the lymph nodes, spreading later throughout the lymphoreticular system and to non-lymphoid areas. It is more common in men, and the curve of the age incidence is bimodal with a peak at the age of 25–35 and a second peak in the elderly. It is very rare in childhood. The malignant nature of the Reed–Sternberg cell is suggested by aneuploidy in chromosomal analysis. Its origin is, however, controversial and there is support for either B-lymphocyte or monocyte–macrophage lineage. There are features supporting both views although at present the latter is favoured.

Clinical features

Incidence in Europe is 3 per 100 000 in men and half this in women.

- It usually arises in lymph nodes, most commonly in the neck.
- Spontaneous waxing and waning of the node size is common.
- A routine chest X-ray may show mediastinal lymphadenopathy, usually paratracheal.
- Mixed osteolytic/sclerotic bone lesions occur and may give rise to pain.
- Bone marrow involvement and bone marrow failure are very unusual.
- Hepatic and splenic enlargement is relatively uncommon at presentation.
- The gastrointestinal tract is rarely involved.
- Presentation may occasionally occur with unexplained fever, night sweats, weight loss or pruritus.
- Alcohol-related pain is described but is rare.
- Infections are often seen and are related to an underlying defect in cell-mediated immunity. Herpes zoster may be seen in up to 20% of cases and tuberculosis is not unusual.

Diagnosis

Biopsy of an involved gland is required to establish the diagnosis. The presence of the Reed–Sternberg cell is fundamental to establishing the diagnosis, but other supporting features are usually present. A histological subclassification is usually made based on features described by Lukes and Butler (the Rye classification).

• *Lymphocyte predominant:* abundant lymphocytes are present with only occasional Reed–Sternberg cells. Lymph node architecture may be relatively preserved. Prognosis tends to be favourable. Incidence 5–10%.

• *Nodular sclerosis:* nodularity is present due to bands of fibrous tissue. Moderate numbers of lymphocytes and plasma cells are present with frequent 'lacunar' Reed–Sternberg cells. This type is particularly seen in young women and often causes massive mediastinal enlargement. Incidence 60%.

• *Mixed cellularity:* moderate numbers of lymphocytes, plasma cells and granulocytes are seen with Reed–Sternberg cells readily identified. Incidence 30%.

• *Lymphocyte depleted:* numerous Reed–Sternberg cells are present often with bizarre appearance. Stromal cells and lymphocytes are depleted and replaced by fibrosis. Prognosis is usually poor. Incidence 5–10%.

Staging

Once the diagnosis has been established an attempt is made to determine the exact anatomical extent of the disease. The Ann Arbor classification is used as the basis for planning therapy.

• *Stage I:* involvement of a single lymph node region (I) or of a localized *extra*lymphatic organ or site (IE).

• *Stage II:* involvement of two or more lymph node regions on the same side of the diaphragm (II) or localized involvement of an *extra*lymphatic organ or site and of one or more lymph node regions on the same side of the diaphragm (IIE).

• *Stage III:* involvement of lymph node regions on both sides of the diaphragm (III) which may be associated with involvement of the *spleen* (IIIS) or a localized *extra*lymphatic organ or site (IIIE).
• *Stage IV:* diffuse or disseminated involvement of one or more extralymphatic organs or tissues, e.g. liver, marrow, lung, bone and skin.
• *Systemic symptoms:* each stage is subdivided into *A or B* categories. The B classification refers to unexplained weight loss of more than 10% body weight in the preceding six months, unexplained fever above 38 °C and night sweats. Pruritus alone is not sufficient for B classification.

Staging is performed by clinical examination and supporting tests (Table 4.11).

The spleen is often enlarged at presentation, but only 50% will be involved when examined pathologically, and conversely approximately 25% of patients in whom splenic disease is demonstrated have no clinically evident enlargement.

Table 4.11 Staging investigations.

Blood count and ESR
Renal function
Liver function
Uric acid
Direct antiglobulin test
Immunoelectrophoresis
Bone marrow biopsy
Chest X-ray
Ultrasound scan of abdomen
Isotope liver and spleen scan
Consider
CT scan of chest and abdomen
Liver biopsy
Barium meal and follow-through
Isotope bone scan
Laparotomy is now rarely indicated as a staging procedure

There are limitations to the accuracy of staging investigations, and there has been a vogue for diagnostic laparotomy with splenectomy and liver, lymph node and bone marrow biopsy. This in general reveals occult disease in one-third of those in whom it appears localized supradiaphragmatically. In this third the stage will be changed and laparotomy may have been justified. However, laparotomy has not been shown to influence survival since chemotherapy is effective in the treatment of post-radiotherapy relapse. Since laparotomy carries its own morbidity and mortality, it should only be considered in patients in whom it may alter the therapy given. In general, laparotomy will only be considered in stages I, II and IIIA where its value in guiding management decisions may lessen treatment-related morbidity by allowing the least treatment necessary without compromising the chance of cure.

Treatment

Treatment varies with the stage of the disease although not usually as a result of the histological subtype.

- Relatively localized disease without symptoms (IA and IIA) has a high rate of cure when treated with adequate radiation therapy.
- Stage IV disease which has extended beyond the lymph nodes usually responds well to chemotherapy when given in combination.
- Patients with B symptoms have a poorer outlook. Many authorities would give chemotherapy to all patients in this category.
- A combination of radiotherapy and chemotherapy is often used in bulk disease, especially to the mediastinum. Selective use of chemotherapy will reduce the area for irradiation.

Radiotherapy. Megavoltage irradiation is the most effective treatment for Hodgkin's disease, and when given to a total dose of 40 Gy (4000 rad) in divided doses over a four- to six-week period is curative. Localized disease above the diaphragm is treated by the mantle technique, which involves irradiating both sides of the neck, both axillae, the mediastinum and upper para-aortic areas. Disease below the diaphragm is treated by an inverted Y-field technique including para-aortic, pelvic and inguinal regions. Long-term complications include:

- Thyroid damage necessitating hormone replacement.
- An increased risk of thyroid cancer.
- Pericardial inflammation.
- Radiation pneumonitis and pulmonary fibrosis.
- Xerostomia and dental caries.

Chemotherapy. Treatment for generalized disease (IIIB and IV) is chemotherapy, and some centres also consider it for IIB and IIIA.

Quadruple chemotherapy using mustine hydrochloride, vincristine, procarbazine and prednisolone (MOPP) is the most widely used, and complete remission rates of up to 80% are reported with just over half remaining in prolonged remission and probably cured.

Mustine-induced nausea and vomiting may be severe, and alopecia is invariable. Numerous studies have demonstrated that chlorambucil may be substituted without affecting the response.

Other combinations such as doxorubicin (adriamycin), bleomycin, vinblastine and dacarbazine (ABVD) have been introduced and are possibly as effective as MOPP, although their place as yet is uncertain.

The major long-term complication is sterility. Virtually all males become permanently azoospermic. Sterility in women is less certain but is age-dependent. The majority over 26 years become amenorrhoeic. This complication may occur less often with ABVD. Following combined-modality therapy there is an increased risk of acute leukaemia at a rate of 1% a year for the first 10 years.

Non-Hodgkin's lymphoma

Lymphomas form a wide spectrum of tumours both clinically and histologically, and are all derived from the lymphocyte. Approximately 75% are of B-cell origin, the rest are of T-cell type. Classically the histological features of the tumours were divided into three main groups of increasing malignancy.

- Follicular lymphoma.
- Lymphosarcoma.
- Reticulum cell sarcoma.

These terms were not specific enough and did not allow detailed clinicopathological correlations. Many attempts to provide a clearer definition have been confused by the lack of concordance between pathologists. The most successful classification was proposed by Rappaport in 1966. His system was based on cellular composition and has defined significant differences between histological pattern and survival in untreated patients. The tumours are designated nodular or diffuse depending on the cytological pattern and divided into three basic cell types.

- Lymphocytic, well or poorly differentiated.
- Histiocytic.
- Mixed lymphocytic/histiocytic.

Table 4.12 Classification of non-Hodgkin's lymphoma.

Rappaport	Lennert (Kiel)
Favourable prognosis	*Low grade*
Lymphocytic well-differentiated (ND)	Lymphocytic B,T
Lymphocytic poorly differentiated (N)	Lymphoplasmacytoid
Mixed lymphocytic/histiocytic (N)	Centrocytic
	Centrocytic/centroblastic
Unfavourable prognosis	*High grade*
Histiocytic (N)	Centroblastic
Lymphocytic poorly differentiated (D)	Lymphoblastic B,T
Mixed lymphocytic/histiocytic (D)	Immunoblastic
Histiocytic (D)	
Undifferentiated (D) (Burkitt's and non-Burkitt's)	

N = nodular.
D = diffuse.
ND = both.

A more recent classification based on cell type has been proposed by Lennert and is gaining increasing acceptance. This system uses the new immunological, cytochemical, functional and ultrastructural techniques to classify the tumours with regard to their cell type.

The newer methods show that nodular lymphomas arise from follicle centres and are of B-cell type. T-cell tumours are especially found in the skin, and many histiocytic tumours are lymphocytic in origin. Two-thirds of the lymphomas are B-cell in nature, half of the remainder are derived from T-cells, and a few are of true histiocytic origin. These are relatively uncommon and are derived from the monocyte/macrophage line.

Clinical features

This group of tumours affects primarily the middle-aged and elderly and is commoner in males. Childhood presentation of the diffuse forms is not uncommon and the disease usually follows an aggressive course.

- Multiple node sites are usually affected at presentation.
- Hepatic and splenic enlargement are common.
- Extranodal involvement is also common including bone marrow, nervous system, gut, nasopharynx, orbit and skin.
- Constitutional symptoms of weight loss, fever and night sweats usually develop late in the disease.

Clinical presentation may be very varied in this heterogeneous group, but in general the disease is widespread. Dissemination is less predictable than in the Hodgkin's lymphomas, but the disease may follow a very indolent course and is often compatible with long survival despite only palliative treatment.

Staging

An attempt is usually made to stage the extent of the disease, which is often disseminated. A full history and examination will usually give the main clue as to how enthusiastically staging procedures need to be pursued.

4.7 Lymphoproliferative disorders

- Anaemia is common and may be due to marrow replacement, autoimmune haemolysis or hypersplenism.
- The blood film may show a lymphocytosis or only occasional atypical lymphocytes.
- The bone marrow is involved in up to 30% of cases.
- Hypergammaglobulinaemia may occur. 10% show a monoclonal paraprotein.

Following adequate staging it is possible to decide on treatment depending on the likely outlook of the patient. Certain prognostic features are associated with a poorer prognosis and require more intensive treatment.

Prognosis in NHL

Cell type	Differentiated	better than undifferentiated
	B-lymphoid	better than T-lymphoid
	Follicular	better than diffuse
	Diploid	better than aneuploid
Patient characteristics		
	Young	better than old
	Female	better than male
	Asymptomatic	better than symptomatic
	Small tumour mass	better than bulky tumour mass
	Localized disease	better than generalized disease
	Untreated	better than treated

Treatment and course

Low-grade lymphomas. This group of lymphomas is generally considered indolent but there are features which result in differences in presentation and outcome.

- Bone marrow involvement is present early in the disease in greater than 75% of diffuse lymphocytic lymphoma and approximately 50% of the nodular variety.

- Rapid progression suggests transformation to a higher grade and rebiopsy is indicated.

Treatment for this group is contentious. Despite aggressive treatment, cure is rare, and the longest remissions are seen in the nodular mixed lymphocytic/histiocytic group (centrocytic/centroblastic).

Stage I and II patients are most likely to be cured, although localized disease is rare. Regional radiotherapy is the treatment of choice although distant relapse may occur, but median survival is up to five years. Many patients with asymptomatic stage II–IV disease may have prolonged intervals with little progression of the disease and require no treatment. In the diffuse and nodular lymphocytic lymphomas the average time from presentation to progressive disease is 8 and 15 years respectively.

In stages III and IV when treatment is indicated there is little to choose between single-agent (chlorambucil) or multiagent (cyclophosphamide, vincristine, prednisolone) therapy. Transformation usually occurs to a more aggressive tumour with increased symptoms, marrow failure and an increased incidence of infections.

High-grade tumours:

- Localized disease is relatively more common in this group than in the low-grade lymphomas.
- The disease is often bulky and rapidly growing.
- Bowel and mesenteric lymph node involvement is common with frequent involvement of other extralymphatic sites such as thyroid, testes and bone.

Traditionally localized disease has been treated with radiotherapy. With vigorous staging techniques a true stage I patient may remain disease-free for long periods following irradiation.

Stage II disease patients, especially those with bulk disease and/or systemic symptoms, fare less well and should receive chemotherapy along with those in stages III and IV. Adjuvant radiotherapy is often considered to areas of bulk disease. Combination chemotherapy is the mainstay of treatment. Complete remission rates varying from 16 to 75% have been reported using a variety of regimens — CHOP, BACOP, COMLA, M-BACOD. No one regimen stands out above the others. If complete remission can be induced rapidly — usually within three courses — the outlook is generally good. Otherwise there is an inexorable progression. Of those who achieve CR, up to two-thirds can expect a prolonged period of disease-free survival with the median in excess of five years.

In the non-responders and in those who relapse, prolonged survival is uncommon and response to alternate therapy unusual. A variety of newer agents have been tried including mitoxantrone, ifosfamide and etoposide (VP16). In those with uninvolved bone marrow, autologous marrow grafting has been tried. There have also been trials using some of the biological immune modifiers — the interferons. These all remain experimental.

Burkitt's lymphoma

The Epstein–Barr virus has been linked to the African type of Burkitt's lymphoma. EB viral DNA and EBV-associated nuclear antigen have been found in the cells of the lymphoma.

- African Burkitt's lymphoma has a predilection for the jaw.
- Histology shows a monotonous sheet of malignant B-cells with cytoplasmic basophilia and vacuoles. Scattered macrophages give a characteristic 'starry sky' appearance.
- Cytogenetic studies have revealed typical patterns of abnormality — t(8;22), t(2;8), t(8;14).
- Non-African Burkitt's lymophoma is not related to EBV infection but is morphologically similar and commonly presents with abdominal tumour in young people.
- Treatment requires high-dose intensive therapy incorporating the sanctuary sites.
- The relapse rate is high, particularly in the CNS.

T-cell convoluted lymphoma

This tumour is a distinct entity. It is usually found in older children and young adults and is closely related to acute T-cell lymphoblastic leukaemia. Most patients present with bulk mediastinal disease or leukaemic marrow infiltration and often both. CNS involvement occurs in a significant number. Treatment with combination therapy usually results in rapid resolution of the tumour, but relapse is usually early and median survival is less than 12 months.

Adult T-cell lymphoma/leukaemia (ATLL)

This is a rapidly progressive T-cell disorder that has been described in two racial groups: Japanese and Caribbean blacks resident in the U.K. Seroepidemiological studies have demonstrated that the disease is related to the retrovirus HTLVI. The disorder is characterized by lymph node enlargement with moderate hepatosplenomegaly, early blood and marrow infiltration and a high incidence of hypercalcaemia.

The lymphoid cells are pleomorphic with irregular nuclei. They have a mature T-cell phenotype, usually positive with OKT4. The outlook is poor.

Cutaneous T-cell lymphomas

Sezary syndrome

Characteristic features of this group are erythroderma with severe pruritus and with a typical lymphocytic infiltration of the epidermis. The marrow is often uninvolved but typical cells are found in the peripheral blood. Lymphadenopathy and hepatosplenomegaly are common.

- The cells are large with grooved and folded nuclei — described as cerebriform. The appearances may be more obvious on electron than light microscopy.
- The membrane phenotype is that of mature T-helper cells (OKT4+).

- The disease is slowly progressive and poorly responsive to therapy.
- Leucaphaeresis may be helpful when the WBC is high and may even help the skin lesions.

Mycosis fungoides

This is confined to the skin and typically starts as a non-specific scaly eruption. This progresses to plaques, tumours and ulcers.

- Systemic involvement is not seen.
- The underlying cell is OKT4+ve lymphocyte.
- Skin biopsy shows typical 'Pautrier's abscesses'.

Treatment is usually local with topical nitrogen mustard, although ultraviolet light and psoralens (PUVA) may help.

If visceral involvement occurs the outlook becomes considerably worse.

Plasma cell neoplasms

Neoplasia affecting the plasma cell produces a group of disorders manifested by abnormal proliferation of B-cells and characterized in the majority by a monoclonal paraprotein reflecting the monoclonal nature of the malignant cell. The immunoglobulin produced is composed of a single class of heavy chain (γ, α, μ, δ, or ε) and one of the light chains (κ or λ).

Classification of disorders

- Multiple myeloma/plasma cell leukaemia.
- Benign monoclonal gammopathy.
- Localized plasmacytoma.
- Heavy chain disease.
- Primary amyloidosis.
- Waldenström's macroglobulinaemia.
- Chronic cold agglutinin disease.

Multiple myeloma

Myeloma is a disseminated malignancy arising from plasma cells in the bone marrow. It is particularly characterized by bone destruction, bone marrow failure and disturbances in immunoglobulin production and is often associated with renal impairment.

- Myeloma is mainly a disease of the middle-aged and elderly and is rare under 40.
- The incidence is 4 per 100 000.

Symptoms and signs arise from the abnormal function and growth of the plasma cells and in particular from:

- Bone destruction.
- Failure of normal immunoglobulin production.
- Extramedullary plasmacytomas.
- Renal failure.
- Involvement of the nervous system.

Bone destruction

Plasma cells increase in the bone marrow so that there may be a diffuse increase in numbers. However, localized deposits occur which may be obvious on X-ray examination as 'punched out' lytic lesions.

- Bone pain occurs, particularly affecting the dorsal and lumbar spine.
- Pathological fractures occur often following trivial injury.
- Hypercalcaemia is seen in up to 30% with symptoms of polyuria, thirst, constipation and confusion.
- Bone marrow failure may be seen due to marrow replacement.

Abnormal immunoglobulin production

Normal immunoglobulin synthesis is disturbed with reduction in all normal immunoglobulin classes. The majority show evidence of an increased monoclonal paraprotein (M protein) although 20% may only produce a light chain. These changes have a variety of consequences.

- Increased risk of infection, particularly bacterial. Cellular immunity may also be impaired.
- A hyperviscosity syndrome may occur with confusion, lethargy, visual disturbance, a bleeding tendency and paradoxically a hypercoagulable state in some patients. This is particularly seen in IgA and IgG3 myeloma where the proteins may aggregate.
- Renal dysfunction due to light chain deposition.
- A bleeding tendency is seen due to thrombocytopenia and the effects of hyperviscosity. However, the abnormal protein may directly affect the clotting factors.

Extramedullary plasmacytomas
Plasma cell tumours may arise in subcutaneous tissue and the retroperitoneal and retro-orbital spaces, and there may be no other features of myeloma.

Renal failure
Some abnormality of renal function is seen in almost one-third of patients at presentation and is especially common in end-stage disease. Many of the factors leading to renal failure are potentially reversible if treated early and vigorously. Causes include:

- Dehydration.
- Hypercalcaemia.
- Hyperuricaemia.
- Renal tract infections.
- Direct renal tubular epithelial damage by light chains.
- Amyloidosis.
- Plasma cell infiltration of the kidney.
- Intravenous urography which should be carried out with care and without dehydration.

Neurological involvement
This may be due to a number of causes.

- Pathological fracture of vertebrae with cord compression.
- Direct invasion by tumour of the spinal cord.
- Spinal nerve root or cranial nerve lesions due to direct infiltration or pressure from extramedullary deposits.
- Hyperviscosity syndrome.
- Metabolic disturbance, particularly hypercalcaemia.
- Infection due to opportunistic infection, e.g. herpes encephalitis.
- Neuropathy due to 'non-metastatic' effects of malignancy.

Diagnosis

The diagnosis may be suggested by the clinical features, particularly when associated with hypercalcaemia or unexpectedly raised erythrocyte sedimentation rate (ESR). A confirmed diagnosis is based on the finding of:

- An increased number of plasma cells in the marrow.
- A monoclonal paraprotein in serum or urine on immunoelectrophoresis.
- Bone lesions (lytic, porotic or sclerotic).

The peripheral blood usually shows marked rouleaux formation and the ESR may be very high. The abnormal protein produces a blue background staining to the blood film. Nucleated red cells and white cell precursors (leucoerythroblastic anaemia) are occasionally seen, reflecting the degree of marrow infiltration. Plasma cells in the peripheral blood are found in less than 5% and more rarely in large numbers (plasma cell leukaemia). Their presence is more usually a response to severe infection.

An infiltrate of abnormal plasma cells in the bone marrow is the key diagnostic factor. Involvement is usually diffuse but may be patchy and can be missed on a single bone marrow aspiration. Malignant plasma cells are usually abnormal with cytoplasmic vacuolation, inclusion bodies and multinuclearity. A plasmacytosis is often seen in chronic infections and inflammatory conditions and may cause diagnostic confusion.

Metabolic assessment should be made with particular attention to serum calcium and uric acid. Renal function should also be measured with urea, creatinine and where appropriate a creatinine clearance.

Radiological examination is abnormal in up to 80% at presentation. Lytic lesions are most common and are seen in the skull, spine, clavicles, ribs, pelvis, humeri and femora. The bones may show generalized osteoporosis often associated with crush fractures of the vertebrae.

Normal immunoglobulin production is reduced but total serum protein is usually increased due to the production of the monoclonal paraprotein. Serum protein electrophoresis will demonstrate this as a narrow band in the globulin region, and immunoelectrophoresis will identify the paraprotein as IgG, IgA, IgM, IgD or IgE with restriction to one light chain class. (60% κ, 40% λ). The incidence of the different types of myeloma is:

- IgG 50%.
- IgA 25%.
- Bence Jones protein only (light chains) 20%, although in 70% of all cases free light chains can be detected.
- A few cases of IgD and IgE myeloma are seen.
- IgM myeloma is very rare.
- In 1% no paraprotein can be detected. The plasma cells often contain cytoplasmic immunoglobulin but have a defective secretory mechanism.

Bence Jones protein possesses the unusual property of precipitation on heating with dissolution on further heating. This technique is, however, relatively insensitive, and all suspect urines should be studied by immunoelectrophoresis.

A paraprotein may be detected in a variety of conditions, particularly the other lymphoproliferative disorders. It has also been described in association with carcinoma and may be found as an isolated abnormality. In this latter state the condition is known as *benign monoclonal gammopathy*. The majority have an IgG paraprotein (90%). This is principally a diagnosis of exclusion but is characterized by:

- The absence of serum or urinary immunoglobulin fragments (Bence Jones protein).

- No suppression of normal immunoglobulin production.
- A low paraprotein level (IgG less than 30 g/l) with no progressive rise.
- Bone marrow plasma cell infiltrate less than 10%.
- No radiological changes.

A small percentage will progress to clinical multiple myeloma (10%).

Staging and prognosis
Survival is very variable and it is difficult to predict prognosis in the individual. Several features are known to be associated with poor survival.

In general the degree of symptoms and signs is related to the tumour mass, and it is often helpful to assign the patient to a particular group when considering prognosis.

High tumour mass ($>1.2 \times 10^{12}$ plasma cells/m^2):
- Haemoglobin <8.5 g/dl.
- Serum calcium >3.0 mmol/l.
- Serum IgG >70 g/l in IgG myeloma.
- Serum IgA >50 g/l in IgA myeloma.
- Extensive lytic lesions.

Low tumour mass ($<0.6 \times 10^{12}$ plasma cells/m^2):
- Haemoglobin >10 g/dl.
- Normal serum calcium.
- Serum IgG <50 g/l in IgG myeloma.
- Serum IgA <30 g/l in IgA myeloma.
- Few or no lytic lesions.

Intermediate tumour mass:
- All patients who do not fall into either of the previous categories.

Plasma β_2-microglobulin has also been shown to correlate with the tumour mass, but its place in routine assessment is uncertain. Survival for all patients with myeloma remains poor with the median at two years. This can be broken down by tumour mass showing that those with least disease at presentation have the longest median survival.

- High tumour mass — 17 months.
- Intermediate — 27 months.
- Low — 39 months.

It is also useful to consider renal function at presentation as an independent variable affecting survival. Mean survival falls to 11 months in those with a blood urea greater than 8 mmol/l after rehydration at presentation.

The type of paraprotein does not correlate with survival although lambda light chains are associated with an increased incidence of renal failure. However, the response of the paraprotein to specific treatment is important. In the group whose paraprotein level falls to less than 10% of the starting value median survival is increased by 6–9 months. End-stage disease is characterized by:

- Increasing bone marrow involvement with cytopenias.
- An increased incidence of renal failure.
- Recurrent infections, particularly bacterial.
- A significant risk of developing acute myeloblastic leukaemia, often preceded by sideroblastic change. Whether this is part of the natural history of the disease or related to alkylating agents is uncertain.

Management

At presentation the patient may have a variety of complications which should all be considered when planning specific treatment. In general most patients will require therapy, but in those asymptomatic patients in whom the paraprotein was an incidental finding there is no evidence that early treatment is of any benefit. Although long-term survival is dependent on response to treatment, in the short term supportive and ancillary therapy is just as important.

- Physical activity should be maintained to reduce bone demineralization.

- A high fluid intake of at least 3 l/day is necessary to protect the kidneys from the effects of dehydration, hypercalcaemia and high viscosity.
- Adequate pain relief is necessary to maintain mobility and may require a mixture of analgesia, local radiotherapy and physical support such as corsets.
- Radiation therapy may rapidly relieve bone pain and plays a major role in the management of spinal cord compression.
- Internal surgical fixation of pathological fractures should be performed for stability and pain relief prior to irradiation. It should also be considered for large lytic lesions in long bones.
- Hypercalcaemia requires rapid correction if renal failure is to be avoided. High fluid intake and diuretics will help most but early use of mithramycin or the diphosphonates must be considered. In the newly presenting patient treatment with an alkylating agent plus corticosteroids should not be delayed.
- Hyperuricaemia should be treated with allopurinol.
- Hyperviscosity can be rapidly corrected by plasma exchange but will recur unless specific therapy is given.
- In irreversible renal failure the appropriateness of long-term renal replacement therapy must be considered before embarking on short-term support.
- In patients with recurrent infections intravenous immunoglobulin replacement may help symptomatically.

Cytotoxic therapy

Myeloma is not curable at present, and treatment is essentially palliative. Alkylating agents are the mainstay of treatment in association with steroids and radiotherapy. The most commonly used agents are cyclophosphamide and melphalan. Both agents are extremely effective and cross-resistance does not always occur, so that if one does not produce a response the other may be tried.

Melphalan is often given in association with steroids as an intermittent oral agent. It is generally given at a dose of 10 mg/m^2 daily for four days and repeated six-weekly provided the neutrophil and platelet counts are adequate. It is, however, irregularly absorbed from the gastrointestinal tract.

Cyclophosphamide may be given orally and intravenously, the latter often as a bolus dose (600 mg/m^2) every three weeks. It is less well tolerated but does not depend on the vagaries of absorption or patient compliance.

- Multiple drug regimens have been tried extensively but several large studies have not confirmed their superiority over standard therapy.
- Second-line therapy with adriamycin, BCNU, vincristine and others is in general disappointing.

New approaches have been tried, particularly in the younger patient, in view of the poor outlook.

- α-Interferon has some effect alone and is now being evaluated in association with conventional therapy.
- High-dose intravenous melphalan may induce a biochemical and immunological complete remission but this does not appear to improve survival and requires intensive support facilities.
- Continuous infusion of vincristine and adriamycin over four days in association with high-dose steroids has produced encouraging results and is well tolerated even in the elderly.
- Autografting following several courses of high-dose treatment with or without an attempt to 'clean up' the marrow is being evaluated in some centres.
- Allogeneic bone marrow transplantation should be considered in the few patients suitable.

Localized plasmacytoma

Solitary plasmacytomas of the bone constitute approximately 5% of all plasma cell neoplasia. Although they are not associated with other features of myeloma they probably do not represent a separate entity but only an early manifestation, as most will progress with time to typical myeloma. Median survival is about eight years.

Extramedullary plasmacytomas may be found often affecting the post-nasal space or gastrointestinal tract. They do not involve the bone marrow although a paraprotein may be present, and they rarely progress to myeloma.

Heavy chain disease
This rare group of disorders is characterized by infiltration of tissues with lymphoplasmacytic cells and the production of defective heavy chains but no light chains.

- Alpha heavy chain disease is the commonest, infiltrating the gut causing a malabsorption syndrome, and more rarely the respiratory tract. Tetracycline may produce a remission but usually cytotoxic agents need to be given. Response is poor.
- Most patients resemble lymphoma with lymphadenopathy and splenomegaly.

Amyloidosis
Amyloid is a protein/carbohydrate aggregate which is laid down in the tissues causing a variety of organ dysfunctions. Amyloid is a waxy infiltration, is eosinophilic and is stained by Congo red.

Infiltration of tissue arises either as a result of excessive stimulation of the reticuloendothelial system as found in chronic infection or inflammation such as rheumatoid arthritis, or because of primary derangement of immunoglobulin synthesis. In the latter, often called primary amyloid, abnormal plasma cells may be seen in the bone marrow and distinction from myeloma is difficult.

Amyloidosis may be immunoglobulin-related or non-immunoglobulin-related; the similarity is due to the protein structure rather than its source.

In amyloid associated with plasma cell dyscrasia the protein is composed almost entirely of light chain and is referred to as AL protein. This differs from the amyloid secondary to chronic infection/inflammation and the inherited disorders such as Mediterranean fever which is referred to as AA protein. Presentation is variable and depends on the type of organ involvement, but frequently seen are:

- Renal failure.
- Restrictive cardiomyopathy.
- Gastrointestinal disorders including malabsorption and dysphagia.
- Neurological disorders including neuropathy and carpal tunnel syndrome.
- Skin infiltration with nodules and 'pinch purpura'.

Treatment depends on the underlying disorder. If following diagnosis no obvious cause is present, myeloma should be excluded.

- Survival in primary amyloid or when in association with myeloma is poor with a mean of 18 months. Treatment is supportive with little effective specific therapy.
- Amyloid secondary to chronic stimulation has a much better prognosis and treatment should be aimed at the underlying disorder.

Waldenström's macroglobulinaemia

This is a chronic lymphoproliferative disorder which is characterized by the proliferation of lymphoplasmacytic cells and production of a monoclonal paraprotein of IgM type. Clinically there is:

- Bone marrow infiltration.
- Lymphadenopathy and splenomegaly.
- Lytic bone lesions are not found and if present suggest the rare IgM myeloma.
- Hyperviscosity may be found as the large molecular weight protein concentrates in the vascular compartment leading to the hyperviscosity syndrome with mental changes, thromboses, heart failure, a tendency to bleed and Raynaud's phenomenon. Retinal haemorrhages are also common.
- Renal failure is rare.

The clinical course is variable and may be very protracted, up to 20% of patients requiring no treatment. Occasionally the abnormal protein may cause problems such as autoimmune haemolysis and cold precipitation.

Treatment may not be necessary for some patients but a low-dose continuous alkylating agent such as chlorambucil is usually given. Plasma exchange should be used if there are problems with hyperviscosity.

Anaemia may occur because of marrow involvement but it must be remembered that there is a large increase in plasma volume due to the oncotic effect of the intravascular macroglobulin and that the anaemia may be spurious due to the haemodilutional effect. Difficulties may arise with cross-matching due to the paraprotein, and inappropriate transfusion may precipitate the hyperviscosity syndrome. Transfusion should only be carried out after considerable thought.

4.8 Disorders of haemostasis

The diagnosis of haemostatic disorders is based on careful history taking and clinical examination (p. 8) before laboratory tests (p. 85) are undertaken. The vast majority of hereditary disorders are due to three diseases:

- Haemophilia A.
- Haemophilia B.
- Von Willebrand's disease.

While acquired disorders are most commonly due to:

- Thrombocytopenia.
- Treatment with oral anticoagulants.

Haematological conditions giving rise to thrombosis are much less clearly defined than those which cause bleeding.

The vessel wall

Hereditary telangiectasia

This autosomal dominant condition causes serious bleeding from the nose, mouth and gastrointestinal tract. In addition, many patients develop vascular anastomoses in the lungs which can cause cyanosis and polycythaemia.

The diagnosis is based on the presence of a family history and visible dilated vessels in the mouth and tongue, but some cases lack these obvious features. Management consists of:

- Genetic counselling.
- Local measures to prevent or control bleeding.
- Iron replacement.
- Blood transfusion.

Attempts to correct pulmonary shunting surgically usually fail, and venesection to control polycythaemia may be necessary.

Ehlers–Danlos syndrome

Patients with this rather variable collagen defect typically have elastic skin and very flexible joints. Abnormal bleeding may occur after injury or surgery and healing is slow. Routine tests of haemostasis are usually normal.

Scurvy

Vitamin C deficiency affects the vessel walls and platelets causing bleeding gums, perifollicular haemorrhages and, in children, subperiosteal bleeding. There is a rapid response to ascorbic acid.

Congenital thrombocytopenia and platelet dysfunction

These conditions are very rare but include:

- Congenital thrombocytopenia with absent radii (*see* Fanconi's anaemia, p. 143.
- May–Hegglin anomaly — autosomal dominant, mild thrombocytopenia with giant platelets and Döhle bodies in neutrophil cytoplasm.
- Bernard–Soulier syndrome — autosomal recessive thrombocytopenia with giant platelets. There is a prolonged bleeding time out of proportion to the thrombocytopenia and a failure of platelets to aggregrate with ristocetin or bovine factor VIII due to an abnormality in the glycoprotein Ib (von Willebrand factor receptor).
- Wiskott–Aldrich syndrome — X-linked moderate thrombocytopenia with small platelets. There is an associated defect of humoral and cellular immunity which results in eczema and recurrent infection.
- Glanzmann's thrombasthenia — autosomal recessive disorder

with a normal platelet count due to a defect in platelet glycoprotein IIb/IIIa. The bleeding time is prolonged and there is no aggregation to any agonist except for ristocetin.

- Storage pool disease — lack of storage adenine nucleotides in dense bodies and encompassing a family of disorders. The main features are a prolonged bleeding time with a normal platelet count and failure of the secondary phase of aggregation to ADP with a lack of collagen aggregation but preservation of the response to arachidonic acid. Measurement of nucleotides shows a reduced ADP : ATP ratio, reflecting the preservation of the metabolic pool.
- Defects of platelet metabolism similar to that caused by aspirin — very rare poorly defined disorders usually due to abnormalities of cyclo-oxygenase, thromboxane synthetase or reduced sensitivity to thromboxane A_2. Laboratory findings are similar to those of storage pool disease but arachidonic acid aggregation is abnormal while platelet nucleotide content is normal. Before this diagnosis can be made it is essential to exclude any aspirin ingestion in the previous two weeks.
- Von Willebrand's disease (p. 271).

Management

Most of these conditions cause only a mild haemostatic defect, but aspirin ingestion must be forbidden and intramuscular injections avoided. With the exception of von Willebrand's disease, treatment, if required, consists of platelet transfusions. For patients with surface bleeding tranexamic acid may be used, and the contraceptive pill may help to control menorrhagia.

Acquired thrombocytopenia due to failure of platelet production

The important causes are:

- Aplastic aneamia.

This subject is considered in detail on p. 138.

- Nutritional deficiency of vitamin B_{12} and/or folic acid.

Thrombocytopenia may be the first sign of acute folate deficiency in seriously ill patients on intensive care wards as macrocytosis may not have had time to develop.

- Leukaemias and lymphomas.
- Carcinoma.
- Myelofibrosis.

} infiltrating the bone marrow

- Viral infection, overwhelming bacterial infection and marrow hypoxia.

Management

Bone marrow examination should usually be performed to confirm the clinical diagnosis unless this is very obvious. A trephine biopsy is useful and can usually be performed safely with a small needle despite severe thrombocytopenia. If necessary platelet concentrates can be given at the time of biopsy.

Any suspicion of haematinic deficiency should be treated with intravenous vitamin B_{12} and folic acid and drugs should be withdrawn.

Underlying causes of bone marrow infiltration must be treated appropriately and viral antibody screens taken at 10-day intervals may be helpful restrospectively.

Platelet concentrates are usually indicated only in the presence of bleeding or to cover invasive procedures, but they are often used prophylactically, especially where the platelet count is less than 20×10^9/l. HLA-matched platelets are useful for patients who have become resistant to random donations.

For patients with surface bleeding tranexamic acid may be used and the contraceptive pill may help to control menorrhagia.

Acquired thrombocytopenia due to platelet destruction

The important causes are:

- Auto- and alloimmune thrombocytopenia including idiopathic thrombocytopenic purpura (ITP).
- Thrombotic thrombocytopenic purpura (TTP) and haemolytic uraemic syndrome (HUS) (p. 174).

- Hypersplenism (p. 144).
- Massive blood transfusion (p. 285).
- Diffuse or disseminated intravascular coagulation (DIC) (p. 285).

Autoimmune thrombocytopenia can be due to:

- Virus infection — especially glandular fever, cytomegalovirus, rubella, measles.
- Drugs — especially quinine, quinidine, sulphonamides, penicillins in high dosage, diuretics, antituberculous drugs, anticonvulsants and heparin.
- Connective tissue disorders. Systemic lupus erythematosus (SLE) is an important differential diagnosis for ITP and a proportion of patients, especially young women, initially diagnosed as having ITP, eventually develop SLE.
- Lymphoreticular neoplasms — Hodgkin's disease.
— non-Hodgkin's lymphoma.
— chronic lymphocytic leukaemia.

These conditions are diagnosed by:

- Clinical evaluation — especially a history of febrile illness, drug ingestion, rash, arthralgia, lymphadenopathy and splenic enlargement.
- Paul–Bunnell test and viral antibody screen.
- Drug-specific platelet antibody tests.
- Anti-nuclear factor and other tests of autoimmunity where indicated.

Idiopathic thrombocytopenic purpura (ITP)

Patients may be asymptomatic or present with:

- Epistaxis.
- Bleeding from the mouth and gums.
- Skin purpura and petechiae.

Intracranial haemorrhage is an uncommon but potentially very serious complication.

- The spleen is very rarely palpable in ITP, and if felt another cause of thrombocytopenia should be sought.

Table 4.13 Clinical features of ITP.

	Childhood	Adult acute	Adult chronic
Age of patient	2–5 years	15–30 years	20–60 years
History of viral infection	Common	Occasional	Rare
Symptoms	Purpura and bleeding		Often asymptomatic
Response to treatment	Spontaneous resolution No treatment required	Good	Poor but treatment not always necessary

- The platelet count is reduced.
- IgG platelet antibodies can be demonstrated in the serum in the majority of cases and antibody may be detected on the platelet surface.
- Bone marrow examination shows a normocellular marrow with increased numbers of megakaryocytes.
- Clinical and laboratory features of other disorders associated with platelet destruction are absent.

The clinical course of ITP is variable, largely depending on the age of the patient and the acuteness of presentation.

Management

Young children require no treatment and spontaneous resolution is the rule.

Young adults with acute ITP usually require treatment and often respond to:

- Prednisolone 1 mg/kg/day. When the dose is reduced thrombocytopenia may recur, when the conventional approach is to increase the dose again before
- Splenectomy is performed. An alternative is to give intravenous immunoglobulin (i.v. IgG) 0.4 g/kg daily for 3–5 days, and this will

normalize the platelet count in the majority of patients, sometimes achieving a prolonged remission where steroids alone have failed.

• Cytotoxic agents should be avoided in young people where possible.

If splenectomy is eventually necessary, steroids, i.v. IgG or a combination of the two can be used to prepare the patient for operation, and younger patients should also be given a pneumococcal vaccine if time allows. After the operation penicillin V 250 mg b.d. should be taken for at least three years.

Platelet concentrates should not normally be given in ITP because they will be taken up by the spleen and rendered ineffective. An exception to this rule is made if life-threatening bleeding occurs when steroids, i.v. IgG, platelet concentrates and emergency splenectomy may all be required. Platelets should be given after the tying of the splenic pedicle. Older adults with chronic ITP often respond poorly to prednisolone and splenectomy and have a short-lived response to i.v. IgG. In the majority of patients the low platelet count is acceptable. If bleeding occurs or an operative procedure is necessary then steroids or i.v. IgG may be useful to increase the platelet count temporarily. It is often necessary to use cytotoxic agents such as vincristine or azathioprine to increase the platelet count of symptomatic patients on a long-term basis.

The management of ITP in pregnancy is considered on p. 310.

Alloimmune thrombocytopenia is nearly always due to anti-PIA$_1$ antibodies which are most commonly found in PIA$_1$-negative women who have borne children or received blood transfusions. The condition is rare because only 2% of the population is PIA$_1$-negative.

• Post-transfusion purpura describes the profound thrombocytopenia which occurs in susceptible patients with anti-PIA$_1$ following a blood transfusion containing PIA$_1$-positive platelets. The recipient's PIA$_1$-negative platelets are thought to be caught up in the antigen/antibody reaction as 'innocent bystanders' and the condition is potentially life-threatening. Traditional management consists of steroids, exchange transfusion or plasmaphaeresis but i.v. IgG has now become the treatment of choice.

- Alloimmune neonatal thrombocytopenia is due to placental transfer of maternal anti-PIA_1 antibody which then destroys fetal PIA_1-positive platelets and causes profound life-threatening thrombocytopenia. It is discussed on p. 312.

Acquired platelet dysfunction

The most important cause of acquired platelet dysfunction is the use of drugs. The most commonly implicated are:

- Aspirin and other non-steroidal anti-inflammatory drugs including indomethacin, phenylbutazone, sulphinpyrazone, ibuprofen and naproxen. Aspirin irreversibly inhibits cyclo-oxygenase and may affect platelet function for more than a week as the average platelet life-span is eight days. The duration of effect of the other drugs appears to be somewhat shorter.

Other drugs which may cause clinical problems include:

- Dextrans. High molecular weight dextrans seem to interfere with platelet function.
- Antibiotics — high-dose carbenicillin, benzylpenicillin and ampicillin and cephalosporins.

Other conditions in which platelet function is abnormal include:

- Myeloproliferative disorders.
- Paraproteinaemias.
- Uraemia. The defect is corrected by dialysis to some extent, and further improvement in haemostasis has been noted after treatment with cryoprecipitate or DDAVP, presumably due to alteration in the concentration or quality of circulating factor VIII.

Thrombocytosis

The causes of thrombocytosis are given on p. 55, while essential thrombocythaemia is considered on p. 221.

4.8 Disorders of haemostasis

The haemophilias

Haemophilia A and B are the commonest inherited disorders of coagulation affecting about 1 in 10 000 of the population. They are both X-linked and are clinically indistinguishable.

- Haemophilia A is due to a deficiency of factor VIII:C and is 5–6 times more common than
- Haemophilia B, which is due to a deficiency of factor IX and is also known as Christmas disease.
- 30% of all new cases of haemophilia have no family history of the disease.
- All the daughters of a haemophiliac are carriers of the disease and all the sons are normal.
- On average half the sons of a haemophilia carrier will have haemophilia and half will be normal.
- On average half the daughters of a haemophilia carrier will themselves be carriers and half will be normal.
- Some female carriers of the disease have factor levels low enough to cause a mild haemophilia-like illness.
- The severity of haemophilia breeds true in the affected male members of a family throughout the generations.

The severity of haemophilia depends on the resting level of factor VIII:C or factor IX as follows:

Factor level (*normal range 50–200 i.u./dl*)	*Severity*
Less than 2 i.u./dl	Spontaneous bleeding into joints and muscles Severe bleeding after injury and surgery
2–5 i.u./dl	Rare spontaneous bleeding Bleeding after injury and surgery
5–40 i.u./dl	Bleeding after injury and surgery only — the likelihood of bleeding being less the higher the resting factor level

Clinical features of severe haemophilia

- At delivery — usually normal. Bleeding from the cord and cephalhaematoma are rare.
- At circumcision — severe bleeding.

Otherwise the child is usually asymptomatic until:

- At six months to a year — bruising becomes obvious as activity increases. Bleeding from the mouth and tongue is common as sharp objects are placed in the mouth.
- As the ability to walk and run develops, haemarthroses of the ankles and then the knees begin, and later the elbows are affected. Hip and shoulder bleeds are less common.
- During childhood frequent bleeds occur into joints and muscles and there may be haemorrhage into the iliacus or psoas muscles with femoral nerve palsy. More extensive retroperitoneal bleeding may take place. Haematuria may be noted, and bleeding follows dental extraction though natural loss of deciduous teeth is not usually a problem.
- In adult life this pattern of bleeding persists, but the frequency of spontaneous bleeding diminishes. Secondary osteoarthrosis and ankylosis develop in joints which have been affected by frequent haemorrhage.
- Intracranial haemorrhage is rare but is the commonest cause of death in haemophilia apart from AIDS.
- Uncontrolled bleeding, especially in the pelvis and around long bones, can result in cyst and pseudotumour formation. Bleeding from the nose and intestine is comparatively uncommon.

Table 4.14 Laboratory findings in haemophilia.

	Haemophilia A	Haemophilia B
VIII:C	Low	Normal
CAg	Low	Normal
VWFAg	Normal	Normal
VWF	Normal	Normal
IX	Normal	Low

Mildly affected patients

Although mild haemophiliacs are usually spared spontaneous bleeding, it is important to remember that:

- Once haemophilic bleeding has commenced after injury or surgery, it will usually continue until specific treatment is given.

Diagnosis

The diagnosis is based initially on the clinical assessment.

Typical laboratory findings are:

- Bleeding time — usually normal.
- PTR — normal.
- KCCT — prolonged.
- TT — normal.
- It is most unwise to rely on the KCCT to exclude haemophilia, especially if the history is suggestive.

Management

A secure diagnosis must be made in a registered haemophilia centre with adequate experience of the disease. There should be comprehensive arrangements for regular supervision in which the following disciplines are represented.

- Haematology.
- Paediatrics.
- Rheumatology.
- Dentistry.
- Nursing.
- Social work.

Follow-up is particularly important for children and those patients who treat themselves at home. A domiciliary nurse can form a very useful link between hospital, community, school and work.

Specific treatment involves the stimulation of any internal resources of the missing factor or the intravenous administration of that factor to achieve and maintain haemostasis.

- Factor VIII has an *in vivo* half-life of 8–12 hours.
- Factor IX has an *in vivo* half-life of 12–24 hours.

DDAVP when given at a dose of 0.3 μg/kg releases factor VIII from tissue stores producing a threefold rise in factor VIII:C. It is suitable for the prevention of bleeding in patients with mild haemophilia A undergoing minor surgery. The effect is lost after the second or third injection as internal stores of factor VIII:C are used up. It has no effect in severe haemophilia A. DDAVP is usually combined with tranexamic acid 10 mg/kg six-hourly because it also releases plasminogen activator into the circulation.

Cryoprecipitate is a crude factor VIII concentrate derived from single donor units containing between 50 and 100 units of factor VIII per donation in a volume of 10–15 ml.

Factor VIII concentrate is a heat-treated freeze-dried factor VIII preparation derived from a large plasma pool, and vials usually contain between 250 and 1000 units of factor VIII.

Table 4.15 Comparison of concentrates for the treatment of haemophilia.

	Cryoprecipitate	Factor VIII concentrate	Factor IX concentrate
Form and stability	Frozen below −20 °C	Powder at 4 °C	Powder at 4 °C
Number of donors	Single donor	Large pool	Large pool
Concentration	Unknown	Assayed	Assayed
Immediate side-effects	Allergy — occasionally severe	Very rare	May be thrombogenic
Long-term side-effects	Viral contamination uncommon	Viral contamination common	Viral contamination common
Potential for sterilization	Low	High	High

Factor IX concentrate is a heat-treated freeze-dried factor IX preparation derived from a large plasma pool, and factors II and X are also present. Some concentrates also contain factor VII. Vials usually contain 600 units of factor IX.

At the time of writing the treatment of choice for

- Mild haemophilia A is DDAVP and tranexamic acid. If the combination fails or is unsuitable then the choice lies between cryoprecipitate and factor VIII concentrate.
- Patients with severe haemophilia A will inevitably need factor VIII concentrate.
- Patients with haemophilia B must be treated with factor IX concentrate.

Very little cryoprecipitate or fresh frozen plasma is now used in the treatment of haemophilia because of the uncertainty that donor selection alone will be effective in excluding contaminated plasma and because sterilization of these single-unit materials is not a practical proposition.

Dosage is calculated according to the formula and tables derived from Rizza and Matthews (1984).

$$\text{Dose required (i.u.)} = \frac{\text{body weight (kg)} \times \text{desired increase i.u./dl}}{K}$$

where K = 2.0 for haemophilia A.
= 1.0 for haemophilia B.

Table 4.16 Desired increase in factor VIII or IX in haemophilia.

	Haemophilia A Factor VIII (i.u./dl)	Haemophilia B Factor IX (i.u./dl)
Minor bleeds	15–20	8–16
Severe bleeds / Minor surgery	20–40	16–32
Major surgery	80–100	40–60

• Factor levels should be confirmed by assay if bleeding is serious or where surgery is performed. The level of factor VIII should not be allowed to fall below 40–50% in haemophilia A or below 30–40% in haemophilia B in these circumstances. For patients on home treatment, doses as low as 250 units for an adult with haemophilia A may be sufficient to arrest bleeding as soon as it occurs.
• If the response to treatment is poor, assays of the concentrate itself and of plasma samples before and after treatment should be performed and a search for inhibitory activity should be made.

Tranexamic acid. Antifibrinolytic agents help to consolidate haemostasis by preventing clot dissolution. Apart from their use with DDAVP they are valuable combined with factor VIII concentrate, especially after dental extraction and in open bleeding within the mouth where fibrinolytic activator is present.

The dose of tranexamic acid is 10 mg/kg six-hourly orally or intravenously.

Tranexamic acid must *not* be used:
• With factor IX concentrate because of the risk of thrombosis.
• In the presence of haematuria because of the risk of pelviureteric obstruction by clot.

Home treatment. Many patients with moderate or severe haemophilia now treat themselves at home. This approach saves time and money, prevents absences from school and work, and has resulted in a great improvement in the quality of life of haemophiliacs.
• Children can be treated by their parents from the age of six years, or even a little younger in some cases.

Prophylaxis. Patients with haemophilia B can prevent the majority of bleeds by weekly or twice-weekly injections of factor IX concentrate (600 units for adults).

Prophylaxis for haemophilia A is more difficult because of the short half-life of factor VIII. Nevertheless, many patients find that treatment every other day with 500 units of concentrate prevents a substantial number of bleeds. An injection is well worthwhile before doing something likely to cause bleeding or before an important event.

Physiotherapy. This plays a vital part in restoring function:
- After joint or muscle bleeds.
- In the management of chronic haemophilic arthropathy.
- After surgery.

The use of weights, splints and hydrotherapy are all valuable.

Surgery. Elective surgery is usually required to correct damage to joints or muscles caused by previous bleeding. Joint replacements are now commonly performed, and good results have been obtained in operations on the hip, knee and elbow.

Emergency surgery is dictated by the clinical condition, but the possibility of haemorrhage mimicking a surgical emergency must be considered.

- Right-sided abdominal pain may be due to iliopsoas bleeding rather than appendicitis — anaesthesia over the thigh due to compression of the femoral nerve is a useful clinical clue.
- Surgery should only be performed in major haemophilia centres with proper facilities.

Inhibitors

About 5% of patients with haemophilia A develop inhibitors to factor VIII, but inhibitors to factor IX in Christmas disease are rare. The development of inhibitors is not associated with an increase in bleeding but, when haemorrhage occurs, it is more difficult to control. The potency of inhibitors is very variable both within and between patients, but the level of inhibitor often rises after infusion of the relevant factor. The management possibilities in haemophilia A are as follows:

- Give large quantities of factor VIII. This is most successful when the inhibitor titre is low.
- Give porcine factor VIII. The antiporcine antibody titre is usually lower than the anti-human titre, and if the former is low this approach may be successful.
- Give 'routine' factor IX concentrate. This is material used for the treatment of Christmas disease and is often successful even when the inhibitor titre is high.
- Give specifically activated prothrombin complex concentrates. These are expensive but they may be marginally more effective than 'routine' factor IX concentrates.
- Perform plasma exchange to reduce the inhibitor titre and then give replacement therapy. This approach is only feasible for life-threatening bleeding or when a patient is being prepared for surgery. In the latter case factor VIII in any form must not be given until the moment of operation to avoid the posssibility of a secondary antibody response.
- Attempt immunosuppression by cytotoxic therapy. This is not recommended in haemophilia A, but see p. 289 for a discussion of acquired inhibitors.

The very rare cases of haemophilia B inhibitors are treated with factor IX concentrate, activated prothrombin complex concentrate and/or plasma exchange as appropriate.

The management of the inhibitor patient is highly specialized and may be very difficult. Treatment should usually be confined to the larger haemophilia centres.

For genetic counselling and antenatal diagnosis see p. 314.

Complications of haemophilia

Hepatitis. Laboratory evidence of hepatitis has occurred in virtually all patients exposed to large-pool concentrates for the first time. Some patients develop jaundice or other clinical evidence of infection, and chronic persistent hepatitis, chronic active hepatitis or cirrhosis may follow.

- Hepatitis B still occurs, and non-immune patients, especially children, should be offered hepatitis B vaccine.
- Non-A, non-B hepatitis is the most common form of the condition in haemophilia.
- Vigorous heat treatment has been successful in eliminating virus contamination in some published series.

Acquired immune deficiency syndrome (AIDS). The use of large-pool concentrates contaminated by human immunodeficiency virus (HIV) has resulted in widespread infection within the haemophilia community. The World Haemophilia AIDS Center uses the following definition.

- A case of AIDS is a person with a reliably diagnosed disease that is indicative of an underlying cellular immune deficiency without other known cause.

By the beginning of 1988 more than 70 cases of AIDS had been reported in the U.K. and patients with haemophilia A have a much higher risk than those with haemophilia B.

A wide spectrum of disease related to HIV infection has been described, including AIDS-related complex (ARC). HIV-related dementia and wasting syndrome have recently been added to the definition of AIDS itself.

HIV virus is very sensitive to heat *in vitro* and there is already clinical evidence that the risk of infection can be eliminated by the heat treatment of concentrates. Unfortunately, no effective treatment yet exists for those who are already infected. Transmission of HIV by normal heterosexual intercourse has been described, but only about 10% of the female sexual partners of haemophiliacs show signs of infection. With adequate precautions the risk for haemophilia centre clinical and laboratory staff is extremely low.

Don'ts in haemophilia

- Don't give intramuscular injections.
- Don't prescribe aspirin in any form.
- Don't allow any invasive procedure without appropriate cover.

- Don't use an indwelling line, especially if factor IX concentrates are to be given. Veins are precious and single venepunctures with butterfly needles preserve them best.
- Don't use antifibrinolytic agents for haematuria or with factor IX concentrates.
- Don't operate without performing an inhibitor screen.
- Don't operate without proper facilities.

Von Willebrand's disease (VWD)

VWD is an autosomal dominant condition which in the heterozygous form causes a mild abnormal bleeding tendency, while homozygous VWD is fairly severe. VWD is due to a defect in the VWF part of the factor VIII molecule (*see* p. 93), resulting in a failure of blood coagulation and of platelet–endothelial interaction.

Clinical features of VWD

- There are usually no symptoms at birth or in early childhood.
- In later childhood common symptoms are epistaxes, bleeding from cuts, and bleeding after dental extraction, surgery and injury.
- In adult life the symptoms tend to improve. Haemarthroses and haematuria are rare although they may occur in homozygous VWD.
- Menorrhagia may be a problem.

Diagnosis and classification

VWD may be difficult to diagnose, especially in mild cases, and the KCCT is an unreliable screening test. Unlike haemophilia, there is considerable clinical variability, but when more sophisticated laboratory techniques are used the pattern within families is consistent.

The simplified classification system (Table 4.17) gives a guide to a complicated and developing field. Types I and II are heterozygous VWD, while type III is homozygous or doubly heterozygous VWD. In addition, there is a very rare form of VWD thought to be due to a platelet defect, rather than an abnormality in the factor VIII complex itself.

Table 4.17 A simplified classification of von Willebrand's disease.

Type	Bleeding time	VIII:C	VWFAg	VWF	Ristocetin aggregation of PRP	Multimer analysis
I	Prolonged	Low	Low	Low	Normal or reduced	General reduction
IIA	Prolonged	Normal or low	Normal or low	Low	Reduced	Lack of high molecular weight forms
IIB	Prolonged	Normal or low	Normal or low	Low	Enhanced	Lack of high molecular weight forms
III	Very prolonged	Very low	Absent	Very low	Reduced or absent	Absent

VWF = von Willebrand factor (ristocetin co-factor).
VWF:Ag = von Willebrand factor antigen.
PRP = platelet-rich plasma.

The key to the understanding of VWD is the appreciation that the high molecular weight forms of VWF are the most important for platelet–endothelial interaction and that the VWF:Ag assay gives falsely high values when these multimers are reduced.

Management

The treatment of choice for type I VWD, and probably for type IIA VWD, is DDAVP and tranexamic acid as bleeding may be controlled or prevented in this way and there is then no risk of the complications of blood product infusion. If necessary cryoprecipitate can be given, but dosage is difficult to judge because the VIII:C level is of little value in monitoring the effect of treatment. The bleeding time cannot be repeated frequently, and assays for VWF and VWF:Ag cannot be performed quickly.

For type IIB VWD, DDAVP may be potentially harmful because it can induce platelet aggregation.

In type III VWD, DDAVP is ineffective because the body has no capacity for VWF synthesis.

In both these cases cryoprecipitate may be used, as freeze-dried factor VIII concentrates are highly purified and have reduced VWF content compared with VIII:C. For consideration of the relative risks of viral contamination see Table 4.15.

- Occasional type III patients develop anti-VWF antibodies and are then very difficult to treat.

For genetic counselling and antenatal diagnosis see p. 313.

Other congenital bleeding disorders

These are very much less common than the haemophilias and VWD and are usually autosomal recessive.

Factor XII deficiency

This rarely, if ever, causes an abnormal bleeding tendency although at low factor XII levels the blood is almost incoagulable in the KCCT test. The PT and TT are normal. Deficiencies of other related contact factors such as prekallikrein (Fletcher factor) and HMW kininogen (Fitzgerald factor) have similar laboratory effects without clinical consequences.

Factor XI deficiency

This disorder occurs in people of Jewish extraction. Homozygotes have a mild haemostatic defect and may bleed abnormally after dental extraction, surgery or injury. As for factor XII deficiency, only the KCCT is abnormal. Heterozygotes are usually clinically unaffected.

If treatment is required FFP 10–15 ml/kg/day is sufficient, with or without tranexamic acid, and a concentrate is available.

Factor VII deficiency
This condition is rarely seen and is associated with only mild abnormal bleeding. Only the PT is abnormal. FFP can be used to correct the defect when necessary, and some factor IX preparations also contain factor VII.

Factor V deficiency
This may occur by itself when FFP is the treatment of choice. It is also occasionally seen in association with factor VIII deficiency.

Fibrinogen
Hypofibrinogenaemia results in soft tissue bleeding after surgery or injury which may be surprisingly mild, even when little or no fibrinogen is detectable in the circulation. All the screening tests of coagulation are abnormal. Haemostasis may be achieved by transfusion of cryoprecipitate which is rich in fibrinogen. Patients with congenital dysfibrinogenaemia are sometimes identified during routine haemostatic screening but usually do not have a clinical disorder.

Factor XIII deficiency
Fibrin stability defects are very unusual but can cause significant bleeding, characteristically from the umbilical cord at birth. Haemorrhage after injury or surgery also occurs, as may intracranial bleeding. All screening tests, save the clot stability test, are normal. FFP corrects the defect but a concentrate is now available, making prophylactic treatment more realistic.

α_2-Antiplasmin
A deficiency of this fibrinolysis control protein has been associated with a bleeding tendency, but very few cases have been reported.

Anticoagulant drugs
The commonest acquired defects of coagulation are those due to anticoagulant drugs.

Heparin

Heparins are naturally occurring mucopolysaccharides which enhance the neutralization of thrombin, factor Xa and other serine proteases by antithrombin III. Heparin must be given parenterally. Possible routes are:

- Subcutaneous.
- Intravenous.
- The intramuscular route cannot be used because of the risk of intramuscular bleeding.
- The half-life of intravenous heparin is about 90 minutes.
- Heparin does not cross the placenta.

Dosage is determined by the indication for its use.

- Prevention of thrombosis — 'low dose':

5000 units s.c. pre-operatively followed by 5000 units s.c. 8- to 12-hourly for seven days or until the patient is fully mobile.

- Treatment of existing thrombosis — 'therapeutic dose':

5000 units i.v. followed by 15–25 units/kg/hr by continuous infusion

Or

up to 20 000 units s.c. 12-hourly.

s.c. heparin should be given by:

1 Pinching up a fold of skin of the abdominal wall.

2 Injecting the heparin 5000 units in 0.2 ml with a narrow-gauge needle held vertically to the skin.

3 Compressing the injected area for five minutes after removal of the needle.

i.v. heparin should be given by continuous infusion following the initial dose. A continuous infusion pump should be used if possible, and bolus injections should be avoided after the first dose as they lead to unacceptable fluctuations in heparin levels.

Control. Low-dose s.c. heparin does not usually require laboratory monitoring, but during pregnancy, when slightly higher doses may be desirable, the KCCT or a specific heparin assay may be used to confirm that too much heparin is not being given. In these circumstances the KCCT should not exceed 60 seconds or the heparin assay value 0.3 u/ml.

Therapeutic-dose heparin should be monitored daily, preferably at the same time each day. The KCCT is the most sensitive simple test and should be maintained at about twice its normal control value. The TT is slightly easier to perform but is less readily standardized so that each laboratory should establish its own therapeutic range.

Side-effects:

- Haemorrhage usually occurs when dosage has been excessive. Drug withdrawal is sufficient treatment in most circumstances but protamine is a specific antidote and may be given intravenously. Dosage may be based on clinical experience or can be calculated. 1 mg of protamine is roughly equivalent to 100 units of heparin, and not more than 40 mg should be given in one injection because protamine has anticoagulant activity of its own as well as a cardiodepressant effect.
- Thrombocytopenia may be due to direct or immunological causes, the latter being paradoxically associated with thrombosis. It is rare in the U.K.
- Osteoporosis may complicate long-term use in pregnancy.
- Alopecia.
- Skin necrosis.
- Anaphylaxis.

Warfarin

Warfarin interferes with the completion of vitamin K-dependent hepatic synthesis of factors II, VII, IX and X as well as proteins C and S. Following the first dose, biological activity is reduced in the order VII, IX, X, II because of the different half-lives of the factors.

- Warfarin must be given orally as a parenteral preparation is not available.

- Warfarin crosses the placenta.
- Effective anticoagulation takes about 72 hours to achieve, and if an immediate effect is necessary heparin must be used during this period.

Dosage is determined by laboratory monitoring but the average therapeutic dose is 5–6 mg daily. It is usual to begin with 10 mg daily for two days, but a larger loading dose does not shorten the delay in the development of the antithrombotic effect and may lead to over-anticoagulation.

Control. The prothrombin ratio (PTR) is used to monitor warfarin therapy and is standardized internationally so that results are expressed as the International Normalized Ratio (INR) whatever thromboplastin is used.

- The therapeutic range for the INR is between 2 and 4.5, but where the commercial Thrombotest reagent is used the equivalent range is approximately 15–5%.
- The INR should be 2.0 to 2.5 if warfarin is being used for prophylaxis of thrombosis, especially at the time of surgery (Thrombotest equivalent 15%).
- Where the patient is still receiving heparin in normal therapeutic doses the PT can be used to assess oral anticoagulation without stopping the heparin.
- Initially the PT should be performed every few days but, once stabilized, blood test intervals may be extended up to six weeks.

Loss of control may be due to one or more of the following factors.

- Incorrect dosage — this is usually due to failure of compliance or follow-up.
- Illness — especially cardiac, hepatic, renal and gastrointestinal dysfunction.
- Nutrition — the effect of warfarin represents a balance between drug concentration and vitamin K status. A fall in circulating albumin level will also enhance the warfarin effect.

• Drugs — the list of drugs which affect warfarin dosage is very large and either potentiation or antagonism may occur. Whenever any change of therapy is recommended for a patient on oral anticoagulants, the frequency of PT testing should be increased.

Self-medication should be discouraged but it is safe to take occasional:
• Paracetamol.
• Benzodiazepine hypnotics.

Alcohol should be avoided or taken in moderation.

Side-effects:
• Haemorrhage is more likely when the INR is greater than 4.5 but can occur at therapeutic doses. Haematuria is perhaps the commonest symptom and pre-existing lesions such as carcinoma of the bladder may be revealed at an early stage.
• Skin necrosis is rare and is associated with protein C deficiency (*see* p. 294).
• Fetal malformation — chondrodysplasia, microcephaly and blindness.

Table 4.18 Management of warfarin overdose.

Bleeding	PTR	Action
No	<8.0	Stop warfarin for a day
No	>8.0	Give 1 mg vitamin K i.v. and repeat after 6–12 hours if necessary
Yes	>4.5	Give FFP 1–2 units plus 1 mg vitamin K i.v. Repeat both as necessary to control PTR but do not exceed 2 mg vitamin K
Yes	<4.5	Give FFP 1–2 units and investigate cause of bleeding

Overdose. Management is governed by:

- The presence or absence of bleeding.
- The degree of over-anticoagulation.
- The importance of continued anticoagulation.

If haemorrhage is life-threatening then a higher dose of i.v. vitamin K may be justified in addition to FFP, especially if there are no plans to continue oral anticoagulation. Factor II, IX, X concentrates should only be given to patients with serious bleeding who cannot be given FFP in sufficient quantity to restore the PTR to normal.

Indications for anticoagulant drugs

Prophylaxis of thrombosis or embolism where a risk is known or perceived, and treatment of thrombosis or embolism.

Table 4.19 Prophylactic use of anticoagulants.

Indication	Drug	Comment
Surgery with risk of VT or PE	Low-dose heparin	Well established
	Warfarin at INR 2.0	Effective in hip surgery but little used
Recurrent VT or PE (including AT III and protein C deficiency)	Warfarin	Well established
Mitral valve disease (especially with AF)	Warfarin	In widespread use
Atrial fibrillation (not due to valve disease)	Warfarin	Value uncertain
Prosthetic valves and grafts Coronary artery surgery Transient ischaemic attacks Coronary artery disease	Warfarin	In widespread use Antiplatelet agents are an alternative

AT III = antithrombin III.
AF = atrial fibrillation.

Table 4.20 Treatment of thrombosis or embolism.

Indication	Drug	Comment
VT and/or PE Arterial embolism	Therapeutic-dose heparin then warfarin	Well established
		Fibrinolytic agents also used
Coronary thrombosis	Heparin and/or warfarin	Still controversial
		Fibrinolytic agents also used
DIC	Intermediate-dose heparin	Controversial and potentially dangerous

VT = venous thrombosis.
PE = pulmonary embolism.
DIC = diffuse intravascular coagulation.

Contraindications for anticoagulant drugs

These are usually relative rather than absolute.

- Non-compliance.
- Drug abuse (including alcohol).
- Known haemostatic defect.
- Peptic ulceration or other source of intestinal blood loss (oesophageal varices, ulcerative colitis).
- Hypertension.
- Completed stroke.
- Renal or hepatic impairment.
- Pregnancy.

The advantages and disadvantages of anticoagulation must be carefully weighed before commencing treatment.

Special considerations apply to pregnancy which is considered on p. 317.

Fibrinolytic agents

Drugs which dissolve thrombi are potentially very attractive in the management of thromboembolic disease but their value has so far been limited by cost and by the risk of bleeding. The latter is due to the consumption of both fibrin and circulating fibrinogen during plasminogen activation so that the blood is rendered incoagulable at the same time as unwanted thrombus is removed.

Administration

Streptokinase is usually administered by intravenous infusion but, especially in cases of coronary thrombosis or pulmonary embolism, a catheter placed directly into the occluded vessel may be used. The initial dose has to neutralize streptococcal antibodies in the blood and 250 000–500 000 units is given followed by 100 000 units per hour for up to three days. At this dosage level laboratory control is

Table 4.21 A comparison of fibrinolytic agents.

	Streptokinase	Urokinase
Source	Streptococci	Human urine or renal cells in tissue culture
Nature	Indirect plasminogen activator	Plasminogen activator
Antigenicity	Strong	None
Cost	Expensive	Very expensive
Risk of bleeding	High	High

not usually necessary but the TT may be maintained at 2–3 times the control value if desired. Smaller doses may be sufficient for direct dissolution of thrombus in coronary arteries. Hydrocortisone and chlorpheniramine are given to prevent hypersensitivity reactions and heparin is started four hours after the last dose of streptokinase to prevent further thrombosis.

Urokinase is given in a similar way according to dosage schedules provided by the manufacturer but without hypersensitivity precautions.

- Tissue plasminogen activator (tPA) has a greater specificity for fibrin than other fibrinolytic agents and its synthesis by recombinant DNA techniques has created the potential for safer therapy with a lower risk of haemorrhage in the future.

Indications

Condition	*Method*
Life-threatening pulmonary embolism	Intravenous or direct infusion into occluded vessel
Recent myocardial infarction	Intravenous or direct infusion into occluded vessel
Arterial occlusion	Intravenous or direct infusion into occluded vessel
Severe venous thrombosis	Intravenous
Blocked vascular shunts	Local

Contraindications and precautions

The same contraindications apply as to anticoagulant therapy but in addition fibrinolytic agents should not be used:

- Within 10 days of surgery, severe trauma or childbirth.

Extra precautions include:

- The avoidance of invasive procedures during treatment.
- Careful handling of the patient.

Reversal

The effect can be reversed by:

- Stopping the drug.
- Tranexamic acid 10 mg/kg intravenously.
- FFP and cryoprecipitate.

Vitamin K deficiency

The daily requirement for this fat-soluble vitamin is not more than 0.5 μg. It is required for the synthesis of factors II, VII, IX and X, and proteins C and S.

The causes of vitamin K deficiency are:

- Obstructive jaundice.
- Malabsorption.
- Dietary deficiency (rare).
- Oral anticoagulant therapy.

Antibiotic administration increases the likelihood of vitamin K deficiency developing for reasons which are not clearly understood.

The possibility of vitamin K deficiency should be considered whenever the PTR and KCCT are abnormal in the absence of oral anticoagulants, especially if the TT and platelet count are normal.

Vitamin K 10 mg should be given slowly intravenously before it is assumed that liver disease, DIC or other coagulation defects are wholly responsible for the abnormality. In the event of bleeding FFP can be given.

For a discussion on haemorrhagic disease of the newborn see p. 315.

Liver disease

All clotting factors are manufactured in the liver, including the vitamin K-dependent factors and those which control haemostasis such as antithrombin III. Activated factors are also removed from the circulation at this site. Failure of haemostasis may be due to:

- Vitamin K deficiency.
- Oesophageal varices.

- Thrombocytopenia — hypersplenism.
  — folic acid deficiency.
  — DIC.
- Reduced coagulation factors — synthetic failure.
  — DIC.

The most useful tests of haemostasis in liver disease are:

- PTR.
- Platelet count.

The TT is only prolonged if the fibrinogen concentration is low or there is dysfibrinogenaemia.

Management

- Avoid intramuscular injections.
- Exclude vitamin deficiency by giving:

Vitamin K i.v. daily for five days. This should be given slowly as anaphylactoid reactions have been described following rapid administration.

Folic acid 5 mg daily orally.

Where necessary give blood product support as appropriate with:

- Red cells.
- FFP.
- Platelet concentrates.

Avoid the use of:

- Factor concentrates — risk of viral infection and DIC.
- Antifibrinolytic agents — exacerbation of DIC.

Stored blood transfusion defect

While red cells kept in modern storage media at 4 °C have a shelf-life of about one month, other elements of the blood are more labile. This is especially true of:

- Platelets.
- Factor V.
- Factor VIII.

Human albumin solution (PPF) is devoid of clotting factors. When large amounts of stored blood are transfused the result is often a haemostatic defect in which there is:

- Thrombocytopenia.
- Prolonged PT and KCCT.

and if large quantities of PPF or crystalloid are used:

- Prolonged TT.

Management

In the event of continued bleeding, consider giving:

- Platelets, which may also be given prophylactically if the count falls below 50×10^9/l.
- Cryoprecipitate and FFP, especially if the INR is greater than 1.8 or the fibrinogen concentration less than 8 g/l.

Avoid:

- Factor concentrates — risk of viral infection and DIC.

There is generally no need to give calcium to neutralize citrate anticoagulant.

Blood filters may be of value but can cause an unacceptable fall in transfusion rate. The use of fresh whole blood is discouraged because of the difficulty of providing adequate donor testing facilities in an emergency.

Consumption coagulopathy

This condition is also known as diffuse or disseminated intravascular coagulation (DIC) and results in haemostatic failure with bleeding and thrombosis.

Causes of DIC

Obstetric	Abortion (especially septic)
	Concealed haemorrhage (abruption)
	Retained dead fetus
	Eclampsia
	Amniotic fluid embolism

Infection	Septicaemia Viraemia Falciparum malaria
Malignancy	Carcinoma (especially prostatic) Leukaemia (especially promyelocytic)
Miscellaneous	Cardiac surgery Trauma Fat embolism Shock Dissecting aortic aneurysm Hepatic failure Diabetic coma Incompatible transfusion Malignant hypertension

Clinical effects

A combination of the following features is seen:

- Pallor.
- Cyanosis.
- Purpura, bruising and bleeding.
- Dyspnoea.
- Hypotension.
- Oliguria.
- Loss of consciousness.
- Other neurological signs.

Pathology

The processes contributing to DIC are:

- Platelet activation with small vessel occlusion and thrombocytopenia.
- Consumption of coagulation factors, especially fibrinogen, prothrombin, V, VIII, antithrombin and protein C.
- Fibrinolytic activation with release of plasmin and consumption of antiplasmin. If plasmin is able to circulate further consumption of

coagulation factors takes place and there is a rise in FDPs. Abnormal fibrinolysis rarely occurs by itself.

- Microangiopathic haemolysis due to red cell breakdown in the microcirculaiton by deposited fibrin. The kidneys and brain are particularly susceptible to ischaemic change in this way.

Death often occurs in serious cases.

Laboratory tests

Because of the fundamental effect on the haemostatic mechanism, all laboratory tests are abnormal in severe cases. However, there is a wide spectrum of disease, and sometimes a more chronic pattern emerges in which compensatory mechanisms modify and limit the findings. Thus only normal haemostatic results in all tests really exclude a diagnosis of DIC.

Management

Patients with DIC are often very sick and may die despite the most vigorous efforts to improve haemostasis. Whenever possible:

- Remove the underlying cause of DIC.

Thus delivery of the fetus in concealed antenatal haemorrhage is nearly always followed by rapid recovery (for a wider discussion of DIC in pregnancy see p. 316).

Table 4.22 Laboratory tests in DIC.

Test	Acute disease	Chronic disease
PT	Prolonged	Normal
KCCT	Prolonged	Normal or short
TT	Prolonged	Normal or long
Reptilase	Prolonged	Normal or long
Fibrinogen	Decreased	Increased
FDPs	Increased	Increased
Platelets	Decreased	Normal or decreased
Euglobulin lysis time	Normal or short	Normal

- Ensure adequate perfusion, ventilation and proper electrolyte balance.
- Avoid intramuscular injections and use the smallest number of invasive procedures compatible with the degree of intensive care required.
- Give antibiotics to control infection as indicated.

Intensive therapy is, of itself, beneficial in DIC.

Although in theory the use of blood products might exacerbate the consumptive process, this is not experienced in practice. It is usual to replace haemostatic factors as follows.

- FFP contains all blood clotting factors, except platelets. It should be given by itself or with packed red cells to restore circulating volume.
- Cryoprecipitate may contain 0.1–0.3 g of fibrinogen and 50–100 units of factor VIII:C per bag. Twelve packs (about 200 ml) will raise the fibrinogen concentration by 1 g/l and it should be used where there is evidence of hypofibrinogenaemia or profound haemostatic failure.
- Platelet concentrates, which are usually issued in multiples of six donor units, should be given where the platelet count falls below 50×10^9/l, a large blood transfusion is required or where bleeding continues in the face of a normal platelet count and despite other measures.

Prothrombin concentrates should be avoided because of the risk of virus infection and exacerbation of DIC due to the presence of activated factors.

Antifibrinolytic agents are contraindicated unless there is good evidence that abnormal fibrinolysis is occurring in isolation from intravascular coagulation.

The use of heparin is controversial and is rarely worthwhile or possible. In theory, heparin should help to switch off the abnormal clotting tendency, especially when combined with FFP, which contains the essential cofactor antithrombin III. On the other hand, heparin may exacerbate haemorrhage, especially where injury has occurred or after surgery. If heparin is used it should be given:

- Intravenously or subcutaneously by continuous infusion pump.
- In modest dosage — 30–50 u/kg initial dose followed by 10–15 u/kg/hr is appropriate.

The use of heparin is reasonably well established in the management of:

- Retained dead fetus.
- Promyelocytic leukaemia.

Acquired inhibitors

Very rarely, patients present with abnormal bleeding due to antibodies directed against clotting factors. The most important of these is the factor VIII antibody. The diagnosis is made by the presence of:

- Prolonged KCCT with normal PT and TT.
- Failure to correct the KCCT defect properly with an equal volume mixture of patient and normal plasma.
- Further prolongation of the KCCT of the equal volume mix on incubation at 37 °C.
- A low factor VIII:C level on specific factor assay.
- Normal or increased values for VWF and VWF: Ag.

Causes of factor VIII antibodies (excluding congenital haemophilia A) include:

- Old age.
- Malignant neoplasms.
- Pregnancy.
- Penicillin.
- Systemic lupus erythematosus.
- Diabetes mellitus.

In many cases no cause is found.

Management

This is essentially the same as for inhibitors arising in patients with haemophilia A but immunosuppression with steroids, cyclophosphamide or azathioprine is more likely to succeed in acquired haemophilia.

Acquired von Willebrand's disease
This condition has been described but is exceptionally rare. Most patients have had myeloma or connective tissue disease.

The lupus inhibitor
This inhibitor is separate from the factor VIII inhibitor discussed above. It is more likely to cause thrombosis than haemorrhage and is discussed on p. 293.

Haematological aspects of thrombosis
Less is known about the factors leading to thrombosis than about those which cause bleeding, and a discussion of the causes of atheroma and vessel occlusion is inappropriate here. Features such as:
- Age and sex.
- Family history.
- Diet.
- Obesity.
- Smoking.
- Pregnancy and the contraceptive pill.
- Malignancy.
- Trauma and surgery.
- Carbohydrate and lipid metabolism.
- Urinary protein loss.

have all been implicated and associated with haemostatic variables without much light being shed on pathogenesis.

Meanwhile a number of laboratory findings have been associated with thrombotic events, some as a result of prospective population surveys and some in the study of patients who have suffered thromboses. Examples of these include:
- Failure of vessel wall function with reduced prostacyclin (PGI_2) and fibrinolytic activator production or abnormal inhibition of fibrinolysis.
- Thrombocytosis, spontaneous platelet aggregation, *in vitro*

sensitivity to platelet agonists such as ADP and *in vivo* release of platelet-specific proteins such as β-thromboglobulin.

- Increased concentrations of coagulation factors, especially fibrinogen, factors VII and VIII.
- Reduction in the concentration of control proteins such as antithrombin III and proteins C and S or increases in others such as α_2-antiplasmin.
- Polycythaemia or even a high normal haematocrit.
- The presence of circulating proteins such as a paraprotein or the lupus anticoagulant.

Unfortunately it is very difficult to know whether any abnormalities detected are due to:

1 A true underlying haemostatic defect.

2 Another disorder in which the thrombotic tendency is one facet of the condition.

3 The consequences of existing active thrombosis.

There is increasing interest in the investigation of patients with unexplained thrombosis, especially those who are young or have a significant family history, and it is useful to have a scheme of investigation which can be applied in these circumstances (Table 4.23).

It thus follows that in the majority of cases of thrombosis selected for further study the following investigations will suffice.

- Hb and HCT.
- Platelet count.
- Fasting sugar and lipids.
- Plasma proteins.
- KCCT with normal plasma correction.
- Antithrombin III.
- Proteins C and S.
- Euglobulin lysis on fibrin plate +/− venous occlusion.

For a discussion of polycythaemia see p. 213.
thrombocythaemia see p. 221.
thrombocytosis see p. 55.
paraproteinaemia see p. 253.

Table 4.23 Investigation of a thrombotic tendency.

Investigation	Result	Value: Diagnosis	Value: Treatment
Haemoglobin concentration and haematocrit	High	Polycythaemia	Venesection Cytotoxics/^{32}P
Platelet count	High	Thombocythaemia	Antiplatelet drugs Cytotoxics
	High	Thrombocytosis	Follow-up cause
Spontaneous aggregation and sensitivity to ADP	Present Increased	Doubtful significance	?Antiplatelet drugs
Fasting sugar	High	Diabetes	Control
lipids	High	Hyperlipidaemia	Control
Plasma proteins	Paraprotein	Macro-globulinaemia Myeloma	Plasma exchange Cytotoxics
PT and TT		No value	
KCCT	Short	Doubtful significance	
	Long	Look for lupus inhibitor	?Steroids Aspirin Warfarin
Fibrinogen concentration Factors VII and VIII	High	Doubtful significance	
Antithrombin III	Low	Inherited or acquired deficiency	Anti-coagulation
Proteins C and S	Low	Inherited or acquired deficiency	Anti-coagulation
Euglobulin lysis time	Long	Semiquantitative only	
Eugloblin lysis Fibrin plate assay ± venous occlusion	Reduced zone of lysis	Reduced fibrinolytic activator	?Stanozolol
Plasminogen	Reduced	Doubtful significance	
α_2-Antiplasmin	Increased	Doubtful significance	

Lupus inhibitor

This coagulation inhibitor has been identified as a risk factor for recurrent venous and arterial thrombosis and fetal death *in utero*. Although often found in patients with systemic lupus erythematosus the anticoagulant is not confined to this group but is strongly associated with the presence of:

- Anticardiolipin antibodies.
- A false-positive test for syphilis.
- Thrombocytopenia.

The antibody appears to be directed against lipid and is usually detected by prolongation of the KCCT, inhibitory activity being demonstrated by the failure of normal plasma to correct the defect in mixing experiments. More sensitive tests based on the extrinsic and intrinsic pathways of coagulation are available, the most commonly used being the:

- Dilute thromboplastin test in which brain thromboplastin is diluted 1 : 500 and the PT performed on test and control platelet-poor plasma. A test : control ratio of >1.3 is considered a positive result. An alternative test uses Russell's viper venom as an activator.

The inhibitor may disappear spontaneously or following immunosuppression, usually with steroids. Oral anticoagulants may also be needed.

- Pregnant women with the lupus inhibitor have been treated successfully with prednisone and low-dose aspirin.

Antithrombin III

Antithrombin III deficiency is associated with recurrent venous thrombosis and is inherited in an autosomal dominant fashion. Thrombosis is unusual during childhood and particularly follows surgery, pregnancy or the use of the contraceptive pill.

Biological assays are preferable to immunological assays because some cases have an abnormal functional protein rather than a lack of the entire molecule.

The normal range is 0.8–1.2 u/ml (80–120%) and thrombosis

may occur at levels below 0.7 u/ml. Patients are usually given long-term oral anticoagulants. During an acute episode of thrombosis heparin dosage may need to be higher than usual, and the use of FFP or antithrombin III concentrate should be considered to provide the missing heparin cofactor.

The management of pregnancy is considered on p. 319.

Other causes of a low antithrombin III level include:

- Heparin treatment.
- DIC
- Nephrotic syndrome.
- Liver disease.
- Surgery, pregnancy and the contraceptive pill.

Protein C deficiency

This produces a clinical picture similar to that of antithrombin III deficiency and the same comments on the value of biological assays, the normal range and value of oral anticoagulants apply.

- Homozygous protein C deficiency usually results in neonatal death from widespread thrombosis.
- Skin necrosis following warfarin therapy is characteristic of protein C deficiency.
- Protein C is reduced in DIC.

Fibrinolysis

Some patients with a thrombotic tendency have reduced fibrinolytic activator which may become more obvious following stimulation by venous occlusion. This is a rather ill-defined phenomenon but is of some importance as attempts have been made to 'correct' the abnormality using the anabolic steroid stanozolol.

Thrombotic thrombocytopenic purpura and *paroxysmal nocturnal haemoglobinuria* are discussed on pp. 175 & 177.

4.9 Some haematological disorders of pregnancy

Deficiency anaemia

The blood volume increases during pregnancy from the later part of the first trimester. The plasma volume, however, increases out of proportion to the red cell mass so that although the total oxygen-carrying capacity of the blood increases the haemoglobin concentration falls. This has been termed the 'physiological anaemia' of pregnancy in which:

- The red cell mass expands by 20% to a maximum at term.
- Plasma volume expands by up to 50% and is stable at 34 weeks.
- Total Hb increases by 85 g but concentration falls by 1–2 g/dl.
- No treatment is required unless a true anaemia is demonstrated.

If the Hb is less than 12 g/dl at booking or 10 g/dl at 32 weeks there is probably an additional cause for anaemia.

Anaemia develops in pregnancy because of the needs of the fetus. The developing fetus preferentially takes haematinics from the mother.

Iron-deficiency anaemia

This is the commonest form of anaemia in Western Europe affecting between 15 and 30% of pregnancies. Most women enter pregnancy with depleted iron stores due to a combination of menstrual blood loss and inadequate intake excacerbated by previous pregnancy. In the lower socio-economic groups anaemia is more common, and in the tropics, where hookworm infestation is prevalent, considerable blood loss in the stool may also occur.

Iron stores in the adult male are about 1 g but are usually less in the female.

Iron requirements in pregnancy may be up to 1.5 g made up of:

• Normal iron losses	280 mg
• Expansion of red cell mass	570 mg
• Iron transferred to the fetus	200–370 mg
• Iron content of the placenta and cord	30–170 mg
• Blood loss at delivery	100–250 mg

4.9 Some haematological disorders of pregnancy

- Lactation for six months 100–180 mg

To set against this:

- No menstrual loss for 15 months 240–480 mg
- The red cell mass iron is re-utilized 570 mg

The increased demand for iron affects iron metabolism so that

- Serum iron falls by 30% (NR 13–32 μmol/1).
- Total iron binding capacity rises by 60–100% (NR 47–70 μmol/l)

and the normal criteria for diagnosing iron deficiency no longer apply. Diagnosis depends on a combination of:

- Haemoglobin level.
- Reduced MCHC
- Hypochromic and microcytic red cells.

Iron-deficiency anaemia commonly develops in mid-trimester.

Treatment. Unless delivery is imminent or anaemia is very severe, oral iron supplements may be given. Absorption is increased and oral iron is usually well tolerated, safe and effective. Ferrous salts should be given to provide 100 mg of elemental iron per day in the form of:

- ferrous sulphate 200 mg t.o.s.

This will produce a response in the haemoglobin level of 0.1–0.2 g/dl/day. Once the Hb level has become normal iron supplements should be continued for three months to replenish iron stores. If the patient cannot tolerate oral iron, if the anaemia is severe or if the patient is in the final trimester, iron may be given parenterally.

Prophylaxis. It has become customary in many hospitals to give iron supplements routinely to all pregnant women. However, if the haemoglobin level is greter than 12 g/dl at booking or 10 g/dl at 32 weeks, this is wasteful and expensive.

Megaloblastic anaemia

This is relatively uncommon in Europe, affecting 1–2% of pregnant women. It is virtually always due to folic acid deficiency as pregnancy does not occur in untreated B_{12} deficiency and B_{12} requirements in pregnancy are small.

Folic acid and deficiency in pregnancy

Deficiency most commonly occurs in *the final trimester* when fetal needs are greater.

- Normal daily requirement = 100–200 μg daily.
- Body stores = 10–12 mg (three months' supply)
- *Additional daily requirements in pregnancy* = 200 μg daily.

Because of the increased requirement the serum folate often falls without a true deficiency. The red cell folate remains stable and normal.

Most megaloblastic anaemia is diagnosed late in pregnancy and can develop acutely, especially when associated with infection. Thrombocytopenia often develops in this situation without prominent red cell changes. After delivery blood loss may exacerbate the anaemia.

Folic acid deficiency is exacerbated if there is an increased demand due to additional factors including:

- Multiple pregnancies.
- Haemoglobinopathy.
- Phenytoin therapy in epilepsy.

Treatment is with oral folic acid 5 mg daily. However, if there is evidence of malabsorption parenteral therapy should be given.

Prophylactic treatment should be reserved for the at-risk population and those with macrocytosis at booking rather than be given to all.

Vitamin B_{12} deficiency in pregnancy

In severe B_{12} deficiency conception is unlikely. During pregnancy there is preferential transfer of B_{12} to the fetus, and although 5% of women develop low serum levels these are not clinically significant.

- Normal daily requirement = 2–3 μg.
- Normal body stores = 3000 μg.
- Fetal requirements = 50 μg.

Haemoglobinopathies

Thalassaemia

Homozygous *β-thalassaemia major* is incompatible with conception and pregnancy. As many patients are now surviving into early adult life and getting married they need sympathetic and careful psychological support.

β-Thalassaemia trait is compatible with normal fertility. With the stress of pregnancy red cell survival may fall dramatically, particularly in association with additional dietary deficiencies, and temporary transfusion support may be necessary. These patients tend to be iron overloaded due to increased gastrointestinal iron absorption, and iron supplementation is strictly contraindicated unless specific deficiency can be proved.

It is particularly important that all pregnant women from areas where thalassaemia is found are screened at booking. This includes all those from the Mediterranean area and the Indian subcontinent. If the HbA_2 level is increased (>3%) in the absence of iron deficiency, this is diagnostic. In this case the partner should be screened as rapidly as possible so that genetic counselling and possible antenatal diagnosis can be offered. If this has not been possible then the 'at-risk' neonate should be followed until the diagnosis has been excluded or confirmed. As the disorder affects β-globin chain synthesis the newborn child is healthy and will not develop symptoms until at least three months of age.

α-Thalassaemia. The position with α-thalassaemia in which α-globin chain production is affected is similar to that of the β variant except that four genes control α-chain production.

- One and two gene deletions produce a mild hypochromic, microcytic anaemia and are unaffected by pregnancy. There is no simple screening test.
- Three gene deletions (haemoglobin H disease) produce a mild anaemia (approximately 9 g/dl) due to reduced red cell survival. There may be quite a marked drop during pregnancy. This may be diagnosed by the presence of HbH (β_4) on haemoglobin electrophoresis or by HbH preparation.
- Four gene deletions (Hb Bart's hydrops fetalis syndrome) is incompatible with life due to total absence of α-chains. In general it is associated with miscarriage of a non-viable fetus late in pregnancy.

Sickle cell disease (haemoglobin SS)
Fertility is not lowered in HbSS and the incidence of abortion is not increased. However, there is a considerable increase in maternal morbidity and mortality. The main danger is from 'sickling' crises which are particularly exacerbated later in pregnancy when the enlarging uterus causes compression of the lung bases. Haemolytic crises also occur and are often complicated by folic acid deficiency.

Management is subject to some controversy but most authorities recommend exchange transfusion to maintain the haemoglobin S level below 20%. Prolonged labour and delivery should be avoided with active intervention if necessary. Anoxia, dehydration and acidosis should be avoided at all times. The transfusion regime should be maintained through the puerperium to at least three months after delivery.

Sickle cell trait (haemoglobin AS)
Hb AS is compatible with a normal life and pregnancy: however, a sickling crisis may be provoked if delivery is prolonged and in the puerperium. The condition should be recognized so that genetic counselling can be offered.

4.9 Some haematological disorders of pregnancy

Haemoglobin SC

Patients are much less prone to sickling than those with Hb SS, but thrombotic episodes do occur and pulmonary complications are particularly prominent later in pregnancy. Exchange transfusion should be offered.

Haemoglobin E

This is most common in people from South-East Asia and is becoming more frequent in the U.K. The trait is symptomless and the disease causes only a mild haemolytic anaemia. In pregnancy it may provoke a refractory megaloblastic anaemia and if the fetus is affected haemolysis can occur *in utero* with the birth of a hydropic stillborn baby. The findings resemble haemolytic disease of the newborn.

Genetic counselling and antenatal diagnosis

If both partners have been screened and are found to carry an abnormal gene antenatal diagnosis can be offered following genetic counselling.

Diagnosis in the fetus can be made by globin chain synthesis studies of fetal blood obtained by fetoscopy in the second trimester. The error rate is less than 1% with fetal loss at under 5%. The time at which sufficient fetal blood can be obtained and the length of analysis means that termination has to take place distressingly late. The advent of recombinant DNA techniques has meant that many haemoglobinopathies can be recognized from cells in amniotic fluid or from chorionic villi.

This approach is based on the detection of alterations in the structure of DNA or on the demonstration of a polymorphic site within or close to the faulty gene. The advantage is that any fetal cell, whatever its origin, will have the gene or genetic defect marker, and analysis can occur at as early as 8–12 weeks' gestation. The tests take only a matter of days and termination can occur early in pregnancy. The major disadvantage however is that the molecular diversity of the thalassaemia mutations means that no one method can be used for all forms. All the methods depend on the use of restriction endonucleases that cut DNA at specific sites to produce discrete fragments, some of which may contain the gene in question. Abnormal genes can be identified if the mutation affects a specific cleavage site, but only some forms of thalassaemia have been amenable to this approach. However, by using family studies it may be possible to extend this technique to the clinically more important β-thalassaemias.

Haemolytic disease of the newborn (HDN)

HDN is due to the passage of maternal IgG antibodies through the placenta into the fetal circulation where they react with the appropriate fetal red cell antigen causing cell destruction.

If the mother is exposed to incompatible fetal cells she is likely to produce an antibody which can cross the placenta during that or subsequent pregnancies and affect the fetus.

- IgG antibodies are produced by immune stimulation and will cross the placenta but IgM antibodies are too large to do this.
- Maternal sensitization usually occurs during labour and at delivery due to leakage of fetal blood into the maternal circulation.
- Sensitization may also occur during pregnancy if there is some form of manipulation, e.g. amniocentesis, external cephalic version.
- Termination of pregnancy at as early as 15 weeks may cause sensitization.
- Previous incompatible blood transfusion may cause sensitization.
- If the fetus' ABO group is incompatible with the mother, any fetal blood which leaks through the placenta is rapidly destroyed and is unlikely to stimulate antibody production.
- Anti-D is responsible for 90% of serious HDN, either alone or in combination with other rhesus antigens, in particular anti-c and anti-E.
- Immune anti-A and anti-B rarely cause significant disease.
- Non-ABO and -Rh antibodies are becoming increasingly impor-

tant with gradual reduction in anti-D related disease — particularly anti-Kell, anti-Duffy and anti-Kidd.

- Lewis antibodies may be detected in up to 20% of pregnancies but are purely IgM and do not cause HDN.

ABO HDN

ABO incompatibility occurs in almost 20% of pregnancies, but the clinically important group O mother with an A or B fetus occurs in only 15%. Despite these large potential numbers the clinical problem is slight. Only 0.1% of infants are affected and only 1–2 infants die each year in the perinatal period.

ABO haemolytic disease is found as frequently in the first pregnancy as later. Once IgG anti-A and -B has been formed, subsequent children, although ABO-incompatible, may not be affected. The reasons for this are twofold:

- The A and B antigens are not as well developed in the infant as in adults.
- A and B antigens are also found in plasma and on other cells and these extra-erythrocytic sites mop up a significant fraction of antibody.

It is doubtful whether ABO HDN ever causes late intrauterine death or a hydropic infant and aggressive antenatal studies are not indicated unless there has been a previous intrauterine death (IUD) for which there is no other explanation.

Rhesus (D) HDN

In the rhesus system antibodies form much more readily against D antigen so the greatest incidence of HDN is in Rh-negative mothers with Rh-positive children.

- The incidence of affected infants with Rh HDN is 0.5–0.75% of all births although with prophylaxis this number is falling.
- In the U.K. 85% of the population is Rh-positive; 13% of marriages have a D-negative mother and a D-positive father and 75% of children will be D-positive.

• The incidence of Rh positivity varies throughout the world.

	Rh-positive (%)
North India	90
South India	95
China/S.E. Asia	99
U.S.A./U.K.	85

This has major implications in considering a problem pregnancy.

• Of the at-risk pregnancies, 20% will be sensitized by the first pregnancy if prophylaxis is not given.

• Rhesus HDN will not affect the first pregnancy unless there has been previous sensitization by abortion or transfusion.

• Unlike ABO HDN, all subsequent Rh-incompatible pregnancies will be equally or more severely affected.

• The majority of affected infants will require treatment.

Antenatal assessment — maternal

• ABO and Rh (D) groups and an antibody screen should be done at booking.

• Particular care should be taken of all Rh- negative mothers and those who have had a previous transfusion, unexplained stillbirth or a jaundiced or anaemic infant.

• Antibodies occur rarely during the first pregnancy ($<1\%$) but the serum should be screened at least at 28 weeks.

• Antibodies are much more common during the second at-risk pregnancy (20%) and rescreening should occur at 20 weeks and 2–3 times during the third trimester.

• If an antibody is found, subsequent action depends on the type and strength of the antibody, the stage of pregnancy and assessment of the fetus.

• A titre of 1 in 32 by indirect antiglobulin techniques is an indication to proceed to amniocentesis.

Antenatal assessment — fetal

• Paternal phenotype — the probability of an affected fetus can be determined by assessing whether the father is homozygous or heterozygous for the target antigen.

• HDN is likely to occur if antibodies develop or there is a steady rise in the titre during pregnancy.

• Amniocentesis may be performed from 18 weeks onward and will provide amniotic fluid to measure the level of antibodies and the level of bilirubin. Later in pregnancy the lecithin–sphingomyelin ratio can be calculated as an indication of the likelihood of respiratory distress if premature delivery is undertaken.

• Fetal blood sampling for phenotyping may occasionally be obtained by fetoscopy.

Amniocentesis. Fluid is normally colourless but during haemolytic disease may become bright yellow due to the presence of bile pigment. The amount can be assessed by measuring the increase in optical density at a wavelength of 450 nanometres. Liley has produced a chart which relates the increased OD to the length of gestation and the predicted severity of the haemolytic process (Fig. 4.5).

Assessment of severity of HDN at birth

At birth a cord sample should be taken for haemoglobin, serum, bilirubin and a direct antiglobulin test. Exchange transfusion should be considered if:

- The cord Hb is 14.8 g/dl or less.
- Cord bilirubin is 85 μmol/l or more.
- In the small-for-dates baby if the Hb and bilirubin are borderline.

Mild haemolytic disease of the newborn

The haemoglobin is reduced from normal but does not fall to 15 g/dl. Jaundice is usually absent and prognosis is excellent.

Erythroblastosis fetalis

Nucleated red blood cells are found in the peripheral blood in addition to polychromasia and reticulocytosis. This indicates a slightly more intense haemolysis and is the name often given to the disease in general.

Icterus gravis neonatorum

The baby may be well at birth but is anaemic (<14 g/dl). Jaundice appears within the first 24 hours and the bilirubin level rapidly exceeds 170 μmol/l.

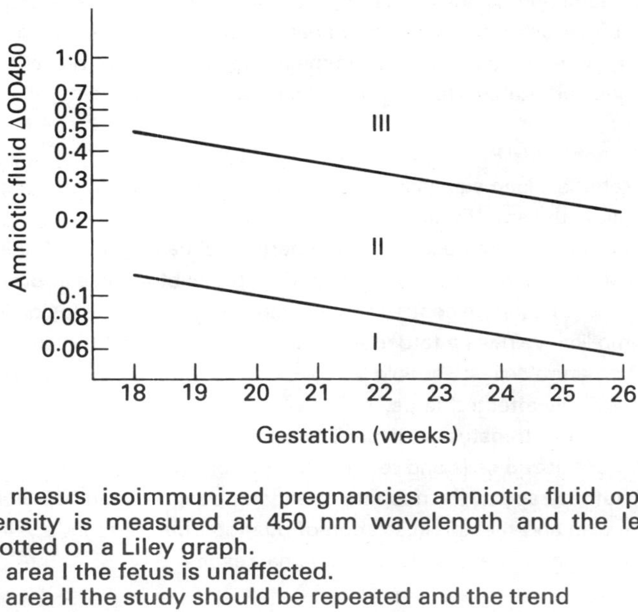

In rhesus isoimmunized pregnancies amniotic fluid optical density is measured at 450 nm wavelength and the levels plotted on a Liley graph.
In area I the fetus is unaffected.
In area II the study should be repeated and the trend determined.
In area III the fetus is likely to be severely affected and action depends on the gestation.
- before 31–32 weeks intrauterine transfusion is indicated
- after 35–36 weeks delivery is indicated
- between these gestational ages action depends on fetal lung maturity determined by the lecithin/sphingomyelin ratio.

Fig. 4.5 Liley chart for an antenatal assessment of HDN.

Kernicterus indicates the neurological complications that arise with the increasing bilirubin level. These are common when the level reaches 340 μmol/l. The infant may die, but if it survives there will be damage to the basal ganglia and spasticity, mental retardation and deafness.

Hydrops fetalis

The haemolytic process outstrips erythropoiesis, and intrauterine death may occur from anaemic heart failure. The infant has gross pallor, oedema, ascites, hepatosplenomegaly and the placenta is swollen and friable. Death often occurs despite treatment.

Treatment of HDN

- Maternal plasma exchange has been recommended in an attempt to reduce the anti-Rh titre.
- Intrauterine transfusion into the peritoneal cavity of the fetus of red cells that are compatible with the maternal blood has improved prognosis. In certain centres the technique of direct transfusion into an umbilical vein via a fetoscope has greatly improved the outlook.
- Premature delivery should be considered from 28 weeks onward in a severely affected fetus.
- Exchange transfusion if performed soon after delivery will remove sensitized cells and reduce the bilirubin level.
- Phototherapy to the neonate to augment degradation of bilirubin in the skin and the administration of phenobarbitone to induce liver enzymes have been used with marginal results.

Prophylaxis for rhesus HDN

Administration of anti-D to rhesus-negative women at the time of delivery reduces the risk of sensitization and in an MRC trial in 1969 development of anti-D fell by a factor of 10. Infant mortality due to HDN fell from 242 in 1969 (0.3 per 100 livebirths) and to 75 in 1974 (0.12 per 100 livebirths).

- It is now recommended that all non-sensitized rhesus-negative women receive 100 μg of anti-D within 72 hours of delivery.

- Anti-D should also be given following abortion, amniocentesis or external manipulation of the Rh-negative mother.

Failure of prophylaxis occurs because of:

- Antenatal sensitization.
- Failure of administration.
- Inadequate dosage.

A *Kleihauer test* should be performed whenever anti-D is given. This utilizes the resistance of fetal haemoglobin to acid conditions compared with adult haemoglobin so that the size of the feto-maternal bleed can be assessed and the dose increased accordingly.

With the reducing incidence of HDN and the move toward shorter hospital stays, an increasing number of failures are due to non-administration. This could be avoided if all the Rh-negative women were immunized antenatally.

Differential diagnosis of HDN

- Any cause of anaemia, jaundice or oedema.
- In particular any hereditary haemolytic anaemia should be excluded especially hereditary spherocytosis, glucose-6-phosphate dehydrogenase deficiency and thalassaemia.
- Perinatal infections, particularly cytomegalovirus.
- Overdosage with vitamin K.
- Galactosaemia.
- Familial hyperbilirubinaemia.

Bone marrow failure

Aplastic anaemia, haematological malignancies and PNH

Aplastic anaemia

A causal relationship between pregnancy and aplasia has been suggested in the literature, although this is by no means proven. It seems likely that the majority of cases develop purely coincidentally. Spontaneous abortion has been reported as preceding rapid clinical recovery, but such reports are anecdotal, and in general the viability and well-being of the fetus must be taken into account along with the potential for haemorrhage or infection in the mother.

The clinical approach is dictated by:

- Severity of the aplasia.
- Duration of gestation.
- Wishes of the patient.

Severe aplasia carries the worst prognosis, and in such patients a search should be made for an HLA-compatible donor for bone marrow transplantation.

Continuing pregnancy and BMT would be incompatible and the possibility of therapeutic abortion must be considered. The decision depends on multiple factors including religious beliefs, the stage of pregnancy and the need for therapeutic intervention. The later in pregnancy the presentation, the greater the need for general support until a viable fetus can be delivered.

Acute leukaemia

The association of pregnancy and acute myeloblastic or lymphoblastic leukaemia is unusual, and the same principles apply as in the previous section. The position is complicated by the need to use cytotoxic agents.

In general, early termination or delivery should be attempted before definitive therapy is given. In early pregnancy it is likely that the use of high-dose cytotoxic agents will produce a spontaneous abortion with its expected hazards in the neutropenic and thrombocytopenic patient. It is preferable that an elective procedure should be carried out with full support facilities. In later pregnancy it is preferable to give less aggressive therapy and delay definitive treatment for a few weeks until a viable fetus can be delivered.

Paroxysmal nocturnal haemoglobinuria (PNH)

This is unusual but occurs primarily in women of child-bearing age. The principal hazard in pregnancy is the associated high incidence of venous thromboembolism. Termination should therefore be strongly considered. Anticoagulation is not attractive when there is thrombocytopenia, and platelet supplements should be avoided as they may provoke a haemolytic reaction. Alternative therapies are of no proven value.

Thrombocytopenia

Thrombocytopenia in pregnancy has many potential causes, some of which, such as folic acid deficiency and aplasia, have already been discussed.

Hereditary thrombocytopenia is very rare but there is a risk:

- Of maternal bleeding so that platelet transfusion support may be required.
- To the fetus in autosomal dominant conditions such as the May–Hegglin anomaly.

Nevertheless vaginal delivery is usually acceptable for both mother and baby. Antenatal diagnosis can be offered to those patients who request it.

Pre-eclampsia and eclampsia

Platelet consumption seems to be the principal cause of thrombocytopenia in this situation, although activation of the coagulation mechanism may also be involved.

- 15% of patients with pre-eclampsia and 30% of those with eclampsia are thrombocytopenic.

Management is that of the underlying condition with the emphasis on control of blood pressure and expeditious delivery. There is no agreement on the value of blood product support but FFP may be useful while platelet transfusion should only be used when unavoidable. Corticosteroids have been advocated recently.

Thrombotic thrombocytopenic purpura (TTP)

This rare disorder has a peak incidence in women of child-bearing age and has some features in common with pre-eclampsia. It seems to be associated with an abnormality of platelet–endothelial interaction which can be initiated or exacerbated by pregnancy and is recognized by the combination of:

- Thrombocytopenia.
- Microangiopathic haemolytic anaemia.
- Renal impairment.
- Neurological dysfunction.
- Fever.

Possible approaches to treatment in pregnancy are:

- FFP infusion.
- Plasma exchange with FFP being given at the end of the return infusion.
- Antiplatelet therapy with aspirin 37.5 mg daily and dipyridamole 100 mg t.d.s.
- Soluble prednisolone at the highest tolerated dose — usually 60 mg daily in divided doses.
- Prostacyclin infusion.

Anticoagulation with heparin is probably ineffective while splenectomy and immunosuppression are unattractive in pregnancy. Platelet concentrates should be avoided.

Patients are often given more than one treatment and a combination of FFP and antiplatelet drugs is useful for the management of chronic relapsing TTP, more vigorous treatment being reserved for the acute fulminating variety of the condition.

Idiopathic thrombocytopenic purpura (ITP)

This subject is considered in detail on p. 258, but ITP is particularly common in women of child-bearing age. In pregnancy it is necessary to consider the interests of both mother and fetus but difficult to predict whether or not the child will be affected by transfer of maternal antibodies and, if so, to what extent.

Mother. Maternal death is now exceptionally rare although a significant number of women bleed sufficiently badly after delivery to require blood transfusion. If the mother's platelet count remains above 50×10^9/l no treatment for her may be required, but if the platelet count falls below this figure or there is maternal bleeding then conventional treatment consists of:

- Soluble prednisolone 60 mg daily, reducing as soon as possible to the lowest dose which maintains the platelet count above 50×10^9/l. If this fails splenectomy may be attempted, preferably in the second trimester. An alternative approach has been made possible by the introduction of:
- High-dose intravenous immunoglobulin (i.v. IgG) which probably acts by interfering with the reticuloendothelial system and is given in a dose of 0.4 g/kg daily for 3–5 days. This treatment may have a prolonged effect on the maternal platelet count but the course often has to be repeated, especially in chronic ITP, and the immunoglobulin is expensive. Its advantage is that splenectomy may be avoided and, for some preparations at least, there is probably no risk of viral infection from its use.
- Platelet concentrates are only given to cover surgery or in life-threatening emergencies.

Child. The following *maternal* measurements have been used to predict fetal platelet count:

- Platelet count.
- Serum platelet antibody.
- Platelet-associated IgG (PAIgG).

but none is wholly reliable, especially as patients in remission, often following splenectomy, may have normal platelet counts in the presence of platelet antibody. Although the intrauterine fetal death rate for mothers with ITP is of the order of 5%, fetal morbidity and mortality perinatally have been very low in recent series. Despite this, there has been considerable controversy over the best method of fetal delivery, which may be summarized as follows:

1 Mothers with a high risk of delivering a thrombocytopenic infant, including all splenectomized mothers, should have a caesarian section.

2 Give mothers prednisolone before delivery in order to protect the fetus.

3 Perform direct fetal sampling during labour to make the decision between vaginal delivery and caesarian section.

- At delivery the infant platelet count should be carefully monitored for the first week of life even if the count is normal at birth.

Treatment is usually unnecessary at platelet counts above 50×10^9/l but severe thrombocytopenia can be managed by prednisolone 1–2 mg/kg/day. Platelet transfusion and exchange transfusion can be added if necessary.

There is growing evidence that i.v. IgG is effective when given to thrombocytopenic infants and i.v. IgG given to the mother towards the end of pregnancy might also benefit the fetus.

Alloimmune thrombocytopenia (*see also* p. 260)
Although it has been estimated that 1 in 50 pregnancies might be incompatible with respect to the PlA antigen system, the actual incidence of clinically apparent neonatal thrombocytopenia from this cause is only about 1 per 5000 births. PlA antigens cannot be demonstrated to be the cause in all cases, so other antigens may be involved, and rather unexpectedly the children of first pregnancies are often affected. Unless the presence of maternal antibodies or neonatal thrombocytopenia has been detected in a previous pregnancy, there are no prenatal clues to the diagnosis because the maternal platelet count is normal, but serious fetal haemorrhage can occur before birth as well as afterwards. Traditional management is based on:

- Transfusion of washed maternal platelets or PlA_1-negative donor platelets.
- Steroid therapy.
- Exchange transfusion using PlA_1-negative blood but
- i.v. IgG shows promise as a more convenient solution to the problem.

If the risk of neonatal thrombocytopenia is recognized before delivery steroids or i.v. IgG might be helpful and

• Antenatal diagnosis by *in utero* fetal sampling followed by injection of PlA_1-negative platelets immediately before caesarian section has been reported.

Coagulation disorders

Haemophilia and von Willebrand's disease
The majority of haemophilia carriers have adequate levels of factor VIII:C or IX:C and go through pregnancy and delivery without difficulty. Levels also rise during pregnancy so that even women who have resting assay values below a figure of approximately 0.35 i.u/ml (35%) are usually safe by the time of delivery. It is good policy to:

- Assay factor VIII or IX at the time of booking.
- Repeat the relevant assay shortly before delivery.

If abnormal bleeding occurs or the factor value is very low then:

- For haemophilia A carriers give DDAVP and tranexamic acid after delivery. Try to avoid the use of cryoprecipitate, factor VIII concentrate or other blood products unless it is clearly essential.
- For haemophilia B carriers consider the need for FFP and tranexamic acid. If essential use factor IX concentrates, stopping the tranexamic acid at the same time.

An affected fetus is rarely harmed during delivery and there is no indication for caesarian section.

The diagnosis of haemophilia in a male infant can be made at birth on a cord blood sample but results can be misleading because of sample clotting. Confirmation should be obtained by a repeat venous sample or by VIII:CAg assay in haemophilia A.

• While factor VIII levels at birth compare with adult values, factor IX levels are lower. Severe factor IX deficiency is easily diagnosed at, or even before, birth, but care should be taken not to make a diagnosis of very mild haemophilia B without a consistently low level at six months of age.

The increase in factor VIII levels during pregnancy also benefits women with von Willebrand's disease, and serious bleeding problems are uncommon. The same principles of management apply as have been outlined for haemophilia A carriers except that:

- DDAVP is not appropriate for von Willebrand's disease types IIB and III.
- Factor VIII concentrate may be too highly purified to produce a worthwhile clinical response.

The management of severe homozygous (type III) von Willebrand's disease in pregnancy may be very difficult and it may be necessary to use cryoprecipitate in quite large quantities.

There are no special hazards for the infant during birth and the diagnosis is easily made on a cord or venous sample.

- NB — where an infant may have a significant haemostatic defect, intramuscular injections must *not* be given. This includes vitamin K which can be given subcutaneously.

Identification of haemophilia carriers

Daughters of haemophiliacs are obligate carriers but other young women with a family history of haemophilia often wish to know whether or not they carry the abnormal gene. The principles of conventional genetic counselling in haemophilia A are:

1 Establish the genetic probability of carrier status.

2 Measure the level of factor VIII:C and VWFAg in the consultand on three separate occasions.

3 Compare the results by discriminant function analysis with the results previously obtained for normal and obligatory carrier groups.

4 Give a final probability of carrier status using the available genetic and laboratory data.

5 Use the information to discuss the issues of parenthood and the value of antenatal diagnosis. It is vital to appreciate that the technique assesses probability and cannot give a definite result.

A similar approach in haemophilia B is much less reliable.

- Gene probe techniques give definite information on carrier status for a significant number of haemophilia A or B families. They usually rely on genetic polymorphism within or adjacent to the affected gene as comparatively few genetic defects are directly detectable. It is important to study the whole family in order to follow the gene successfully, and the possibility of cross-over has to be taken into account.

Antenatal diagnosis for haemophilia and von Willebrand's disease

Early work in haemophilia concentrated on simple fetal sexing *in utero* and termination was offered if a male pregnancy was diagnosed.

More recently, fetoscopy has allowed direct measurement of fetal factor VIII or IX levels at about 20 weeks of pregnancy with termination being offered for affected male pregnancies only.

Gene probe techniques performed on chorionic villus samples early in pregnancy promise to allow reliable early antenatal diagnosis in a substantial number of cases in the future.

As von Willebrand's disease is a comparatively mild disorder in most cases, genetic counselling is usually straightforward and antenatal diagnosis is rarely necessary.

For those patients who marry an affected relative or someone else with von Willebrand's disease, there is a 1 : 4 risk of having a child with type III von Willebrand's disease. The safest policy is to test the partner of all patients with von Willebrand's disease if they wish to start a family. If both partners are affected, antenatal diagnosis can be offered, if desired, using assays of factor VIII activity on samples obtained fetoscopically at 20 weeks' gestation.

Acquired factor VIII inhibitors

This rare complication of pregnancy can cause serious bleeding. Diagnosis and management are discussed on pp. 96 and 289. There is a tendency for the factor VIII inhibitor to decline after delivery and the infant is not usually clinically affected.

Haemorrhagic disease of the newborn

Vitamin K deficiency in the first few days of life is due to a combination of low body stores and hepatic immaturity. It can result in bruising and mucosal bleeding and is usually prevented by:

- Prophylactic vitamin K, 1 mg i.m. or i.v. at birth.

Consumption coagulopathy (diffuse or disseminated intravascular coagulation — DIC)

The principal obstetric causes of DIC are given on p. 285 together with a general account of the subject.

Bleeding in obstetrics can happen with frightening speed and intensity, and serious haemorrhage does not necessarily mean that DIC is occurring. Equally, placental abruption can create profound consumption coagulopathy without any visible blood loss. In general, the haemostatic mechanisms will return to normal as soon as the precipitating factors are removed and the contraction of an empty uterus will independently limit haemorrhage. Management is therefore based on:

- Rapid delivery by the safest route.
- The provision of blood products.

The speed of response to the emergency requires careful forward planning. Ensure:

- Proper antenatal care with blood group antibody screening.
- Adequate access to red cells, FFP, cyropreciptate and platelet concentrates.
- That correctly labelled forms with appropriate sample tubes are available at a moment's notice.

1 Sequestrene tube for routine haematology and platelets.
2 Prothrombin tube for clotting screen.
3 FDP tube.
4 Plain glass tube for blood transfusion.

- That when drawing blood the samples are not contaminated with heparin and that the tubes are correctly filled.

Without waiting for the results of blood tests maintain blood volume as far as possible using:

- Red cells and FFP if immediately available.
- Failing that, plasma expanders such as PPF or Haemaccel in the first instance.

- Cryoprecipitate and platelets can be given later, if necessary, should a diagnosis of DIC be confirmed.
- In placental abruption it is usually best to deliver vaginally but caesarian section may be justified if the fetus is still alive or vaginal delivery does not seem likely to occur without a long delay. Heparin is not indicated.
- In amniotic fluid embolism, respiratory failure and cerebral dysfunction are at least as important as the haemostatic problems but the maintenance of the circulation remains a vital part of management.
- In retained dead fetus there is time to restore haemostatic balance before delivery. Heparin 15 units/kg/hr for up to 48 hours may be given with FFP and cyroprecipitate if necessary, followed by discontinuation of the heparin and vaginal delivery.

The lupus inhibitor

This subject is also considered on p. 293. The lupus inhibitor is associated with a high fetal mortality *in utero* and not infrequently occurs in women without systemic lupus erythematosus.

Treatment with:

- Prednisone 40–60 mg daily.
- Soluble aspirin 75 mg daily.

has been reported to abolish the inhibitor and improve the chances of successful delivery.

Anticoagulation

The usual indications for anticoagulation in pregnancy are:

- Those at high risk of thrombosis because of age, parity, obesity or operative delivery.
- Venous thrombosis and/or pulmonary embolism during the current pregnancy.
- A past history of venous thrombosis and/or pulmonary embolism.
- Antithrombin III (or protein C) deficiency.
- Cardiac valve defects and prosthetic heart valves.

Table 4.24 Advantages and disadvantages of anticoagulants in pregnancy.

	Warfarin	Heparin
Placental transfer	Yes	No
Fetal abnormality	Chondrodysplasia Microcephaly Blindness	No
Fetal anticoagulation	Yes Cerebral haemorrhage at delivery	 No
Oral therapy	Yes	No
Maternal side-effects	Usual risk of bleeding	Osteoporosis Thrombocytopenia Alopecia Bruising at injection site

For those generally thought to be at high risk of thrombosis at the time of delivery, routine low-dose s.c. heparin prophylaxis is a reasonable approach though it precludes epidural anaesthesia. An alternative is the use of dextran.

Established thrombosis or embolism should be treated immediately with full-dose intravenous heparin, and if progress is satisfactory the dose can be reduced and the heparin administered subcutaneously after a few days, continuing throughout the rest of pregnancy.

For prophylactic use heparin is given subcutaneously, if possible by the mother at home, and a dose of 8–10 000 units 12-hourly is often advised. It is difficult to know how early in pregnancy to begin heparin in view of the potential side-effects for the mother and the inconvenience of treatment, and it is wise to monitor the dose by heparin assay at each antenatal visit, maintaining the level below 0.3 u/ml. The most important side-effect of osteoporosis is more likely to develop after long-term heparin administration, and for many women it is reasonable to delay prophylaxis until 32–36 weeks of gestation. If it is acceptable to treat only at the time of delivery, dextran is again an alternative.

For women with cardiac valve defects or prosthetic valves, the choice lies between continuing warfarin and accepting the risks to the fetus or using a comparatively high-dose heparin regimen. A compromise solution is to use heparin until 12 weeks followed by warfarin until 36 weeks and then revert to heparin until after delivery.

In antithrombin III deficiency one approach has been to use a monitored heparin regimen throughout pregnancy to achieve a prolonged KCCT and give antithrombin III concentrate at the time of delivery.

After delivery women who require continued anticoagulation, whether for a short time or indefinitely, may resume warfarin and may safely breast-feed.

4.10 Use of blood products

A transfusion should never be given without a definite indication and an attempt should be made to ascertain the cause of the deficiency.

Red cell therapy

The main indication for transfusion is anaemic hypoxia, when the haemoglobin has fallen to such a level as to cause symptoms or to jeopardize other treatment.

- The average adult carries 900 ml of oxygen in the blood.
- Anoxic symptoms occur when oxygen carriage falls to 650 ml (9.0 g/dl).
- Anaemia occurring over a prolonged period can be tolerated to 4.5 g/dl.
- Each unit of blood contains 66 g of haemoglobin.
- Each gram of haemoglobin carries 1.34 ml of oxygen.
- One unit of red cell concentrate increases the Hb by 1 g/dl and the haematocrit by 0.03 (3%).

The clinical state of the patient should always be taken into consideration, and it is rarely, if ever, justifiable to transfuse a single unit of red cells. In general, blood loss of up to 800 ml can be replaced by crystalloid or colloid solutions.

Grouping and compatibility testing

For the patient to derive benefit from the transfusion, the red cells must survive in the circulation, therefore the donor and recipient blood must be compatible.

- Each patient requiring transfusion should have an ABO and rhesus (D) grouping and antibody screen.
- Before transfusion, compatibility testing between the patient's serum and donor red cells should be performed.
- In an emergency an abbreviated cross-match can be performed in 20–30 minutes but must be followed by a full cross-match later.
- Out of hours' staff may not be available to perform an emergency cross-match and this should be considered in planning urgent, elective surgery.
- Whenever possible blood of the same ABO and Rh type should be given.
- In an absolute emergency uncross-matched group O rhesus (D) negative units can be given unless the patient is known to have antibodies.
- If the patient's group is known then blood of that group may be used but a cross-match is still essential.
- In women of child-bearing age other blood groups should be considered (e.g. Kell) when choosing blood.
- Each request for blood should be accompanied by a form with unequivocal identification of the patient.
- When repeated transfusions are given, immune antibodies may develop and a fresh sample for cross-matching is required if a gap of more than three days has elapsed since the previous sample.

Whole blood is specifically indicated in massive haemorrhage where there is a requirement for oxygen-carrying capacity, volume replacement and clotting factors. Whole blood is usually collected into an anticoagulant solution containing citrate, phosphate, dextrose and adenine (CPD-A). Citrate prevents coagulation by binding calcium; the other components help maintain red cell ATP and 2, 3-DPG levels which are essential for the metabolic processes that maintain cellular viability and oxygen transport. The 'shelf-life' of the unit is approximately five weeks, however several changes occur during this time.

- Gradual reduction in red cell viability with a mean red cell recovery of 70% at five weeks.
- Reduction in 2, 3-DPG increases the oxygen affinity of the red cell (causing relative tissue anoxia).
- Platelets and granulocytes become non-functional at 4°C within hours of collection.
- Cellular metabolism causes an increase in plasma potassium and a rise in the hydrogen ion concentration with a lowering of pH.
- Coagulation factors V and VIII drop by 50% within 24 hours of collection.
- There is a progressive tendency toward clumping and aggregation of white cells, platelets, fibrinogen and some red cells which may cause respiratory distress in the acutely ill patient after transfusion, due to obstruction of the pulmonary circulation.

Fresh whole blood less than 24 hours old is sometimes requested in massive haemorrhage when the labile coagulation factors and platelets are required. As the blood is needed urgently there is no time to check for syphilis, hepatitis B surface antigen or anti-HIV and fresh whole blood is rarely given.

Whole blood less than five days old will be free from most of the storage effects, in particular the loss of 2, 3-DPG. It is preferable in the acutely ill patient and should be used for exchange transfusion in neonates and in sickle cell disease. Haemostatically, however, it is no better than older blood.

4.10 Use of blood products

- Due to the limited supply of fresh whole blood and difficulties with quality control, it is often better to give a mixture of red cells, platelets and FFP in massive haemorrhage (*see* p. 285).

Red cell concentrates are most commonly offered for haemoglobin replacement due to the high level of fractionation of whole blood.

- Plasma-reduced blood is most widely used. The haematocrit is 60–65% due to removal of up to 200 ml of plasma, and its high viscosity may reduce flow if large volumes are required rapidly. Red cells are now being presented in optimal additive solutions such as SAG-mannitol. These improve red cell viability and flow characteristics, at the same time making more plasma available for fractionation.
- Leucocyte-poor blood should be used in patients who have febrile transfusion reactions as these are often due to non-viable whole or fragmented white cells. The blood can be prepared by a technique of inverted centrifugation. A more stringent removal of white cells can be achieved by washing the red cells or using 'in-line' filters.
- Washed red cells contain few white cells or platelets. In addition, plasma is also removed if reactions are considered to be due to plasma proteins.
- Frozen thawed red cells are expensive and difficult to obtain but are used for long-term storage of rare blood groups and for storage of blood for autotransfusion in individuals with multiple alloantibodies.

Autologous blood transfusion

Autologous blood transfusion has been advocated in patients requiring planned operative procedures that require few units of blood such as transurethral resection of the prostate or joint replacement. It will reduce the dangers of transfusion, compatibility testing is not required and there is no risk of transmission of infection from donor to recipient. If autologous transfusion is to be used to any degree it will require a high standard of clerical control, handling and storage. Unfortunately, this approach is not applicable to those patients particularly at risk from multiple transfusion such as those who require major surgery or have bone marrow failure.

Synthetic oxygen-carrying agents

Fluorinated hydrocarbons have been widely studied and are artificial blood substitutes as they readily dissolve oxygen. One product, 'Fluosol-DA', has been used clinically but there remain various problems.

- Batch variability alters solubility and plasma clearance time.
- Microembolism formation or platelet clumping is encouraged.
- Calcium and other cation binding occurs.
- Disseminated intravascular coagulation may be provoked.

Transfusion reactions

These occur in less than 5% of transfusions and are more common in multiparous women and in multitransfused patients. In general, reactions are mild and true red cell incompatibility with haemolysis is rare, being more often related to organizational or clerical error than to mistakes within the laboratory.

Clinical features

Symptoms may be severe and occur almost immediately, as in ABO incompatibility, or develop gradually toward the end of the transfusion, as in white cell reactions. Occasionally the reactions are silent or occur after the transfusion (delayed reactions) and are then often manifest by shortened red cell survival, the only indication being that the response to transfusion was not as good as expected. It is imperative that antibody screening is performed before each transfusion. Symptoms and signs include:

- Fever and rigors.
- Pain at the site of the infusion.
- Retrosternal pain (angina) and breathlessness.

- Hypotension.
- Abdominal discomfort due to lumbar pain and urgency to defaecate.
- Haemoglobinuria.
- Bleeding manifestations associated with disseminated intravascular coagulation.
- Renal failure.
- The anaesthetized patient may show only a bleeding tendency.

Action to be taken:

- Stop the transfusion and monitor renal function.
- Check the clerical information.
- Collect patient samples:

  Clotted sample to verify ABO group and repeat antibody screen.

  Heparinized sample for haptoglobin, free haemoglobin and methaemalbumin.

  Citrate sample for a clotting screen.

  Sequestrene sample for haemoglobin, platelet count and direct antiglobulin test.

  Blood cultures on patient's blood.
- The donor unit should be returned to the laboratory for re-typing and microbiological testing.
- The patient's pre-sample in the laboratory should be re-typed and the cross-match repeated with the pre- and post-serum samples.

Treatment includes

- Fluid replacement to prevent hypotension using blood, colloid or saline as clinically appropriate.
- Mannitol may be given to maintain renal blood flow — 100 ml of 20% solution over five minutes; frusemide may also be given.
- Replacement of depleted coagulation factors and platelets.
- Dialysis if renal failure develops.

4.10 Use of blood products

Causes of transfusion reactions

Red cells. Haemolysis may be intra- or extravascular.

- Acute intravascular haemolysis usually follows ABO-incompatible transfusion with many of the features already discussed. Similar reactions may be seen with antibodies directed against the Kell, Duffy and Kidd antigen systems.
- Extravascular haemolysis occurs due to IgG antibodies, typically found directed against the rhesus system. The antibodies do not bind complement but bind to the red cells causing their clearance by the reticuloendothelial system.
- Delayed reactions occur when an antibody is stimulated by the transfusion but was not found at the initial cross-match. Usually the recipient has been sensitized by a previous transfusion and further transfusion causes a rapid secondary response with haemolysis at 10–14 days.

White cells. Febrile reactions are the most common form of transfusion reactions and are due to alloantibodies directed against white cells induced by pregnancy or previous transfusion. The strength of reaction is related to the tranfusion load and can usually be prevented by using leucocyte-poor blood.

Platelets. Post-transfusion purpura occurs 7–10 days after transfusion, usually in women who have had a previous transfusion or pregnancies. The patients are found to be negative for the alloantigen PIA_1. The condition is self-limiting but may be fatal (*see* p. 260).

Serum proteins. Febrile and urticarial reactions may occur due to reactions to components in the donor plasma, especially antibodies to IgA, which is absent in 1 in 700 recipients.

Anaphylactoid reactions may occur and require urgent treatment with adrenaline and corticosteroids.

Non-immunological:

- Circulatory overload.
- Haemolysis due to — overheating or freezing red cells prior to infusion.
  — infusion through a small-bore needle.
  — excessive infusion pressure.
  — infusion of large quantities of aged blood.
- Septicaemia. Pseudomonas will multiply at 4°C and if the blood is contaminated at collection may cause a severe and often fatal reaction. The risk with platelet concentrates which are stored at 22 °C is much greater.
- Air embolism is very rare with the use of plastic bags.
- Thrombophlebitis is particularly common with prolonged intravenous administration.
- Transfusion siderosis — every unit contains approximately 200 mg of iron. With multiple blood transfusions iron may accumulate in the liver, heart and certain endocrine organs, impairing their function.
- Infections transmitted by blood:
  Hepatitis.
  Cytomegalovirus.
  HIV.
  Infectious mononucleosis.
  Syphilis.
  Malaria.

Post-transfusion hepatitis (PTH) is the most common lethal complication of blood transfusion. Reported cases have, however, declined dramatically over the last decade since the introduction of routine screening for hepatitis B surface antigen (HBsAg). Hepatitis B is now largely preventable, but other viruses have emerged as responsible for PTH.

Hepatitis B, caused by a DNA virus, is almost exclusively bloodborne.

• Random volunteer blood donors in the U.K. have a frequency of HBsAg of 0.1%.

The majority of donors have no history of hepatitis and will have normal liver function. Following infection the virus invades the liver where it replicates, releasing large amounts of surface antigen and small amounts of core antigen into the bloodstream. The e antigen may also be detected during this early phase and is a reflection of infectivity. Once anti-HB_e and anti-HB_c appear, the ability to transmit PTH greatly diminishes and the blood of donors with anti-Hb_s will not transmit hepatitis B.

The most sensitive method for detecting HBsAg is radioimmunoassay. Since the incubation period is variable (36–150 days) a small number of infected donor units may slip through, but the risk is certainly less than 1 in 20 000.

• Hepatitis A, caused by an RNA virus, is only rarely transmitted by transfusion, being almost exclusively confined to the faecal–oral route.

• In a number of large studies the incidence of PTH is up to 10%. Most of these are asymptomatic and anicteric and the majority are due to a virus that does not have markers for hepatitis A or B and is known as non-A, non-B hepatitis. There appear to be at least two different types of non-A, non-B virus with a short (2–4 weeks) and a long (6–15 weeks) incubation period. Although clinically usually mild, severe liver damage may occur; up to 60% of patients have abnormal liver enzymes after a year and 10% progress to cirrhosis. The diagnosis is one of exclusion since there is no screening test. The risk is particularly high in patients who have received pooled plasma concentrates (factors VIII and IX).

• Cytomegalovirus infections are particularly common in patients who receive fresh blood transfusions or granulocyte concentrates. At least 12% of donors have CMV-infected leucocytes, and up to 60% have complement-fixing antibodies. The virus becomes non-viable after storage at 4 °C for a few days. The infection is clinically insignificant except in two instances when a fulminant viral infection may occur:

1 Premature infants.
2 The immunosuppressed patient.

Exposure to hepatitis:

- Laboratory personnel may be infected by contaminated material.
- Exposed staff should be screened for HBsAg and/or anti-HBs.
- Staff with no evidence of previous infection should receive hepatitis B immune globulin.
- At-risk staff should be offered immunization with hepatitis B vaccine.

Human immunodeficiency virus (HIV). HIV infection is the cause of acquired immune deficiency syndrome (AIDS) and can be transmitted by blood transfusion. So far in the U.K. the majority of cases of infection by this route have been due to the administration of large-pool factor VIII concentrate, but the potential risk of transmission by individual contaminated donor units exists.

The safety of blood products is being maintained by:

- Exclusion of donors belonging to high-risk groups.
  1 Homosexual or bisexual men and their sexual partners.
  2 Intravenous drug abusers and their sexual partners.
  3 Patients with haemophilia, their sexual partners and members of the family who help them with their treatment. Those directly responsible for the care of patients with haemophilia should also be excluded.
  4 People who have recently lived in Haiti or Central or East Africa.
- The testing of all donor units for evidence of infection by the anti-HIV antibody test.
- The further processing and pasteurization of plasma products where possible.

Thus the following products are regarded as safe from this point of view.

- Human albumin solution or plasma protein fraction (PPF).
- Immunoglobulin preparations.
- Heat-treated factor VIII and IX concentrates.
- Whilst it is not possible to pasteurize red cells, FFP, platelets and granulocyte concentrates, the risk of HIV infection from these products must now be very low.

With proper precautions the risk of HIV transmission within the laboratory is negligible.

Platelet concentrates

Indications

- Symptomatic thrombocytopenia with bleeding. Transfusion is less effective if the low platelet count is due to immune destruction (ITP) but is particularly useful when there is chemotherapy-induced marrow depression, e.g. acute leukaemia during induction therapy.
- Prophylaxis when there is a very low platelet count. These indications vary, but in marrow depression platelet supplements are usually given when the count is $<20 \times 10^9$/l. If surgery is considered supplements should be given if the count is $<75 \times 10^9$/l.
- Bleeding associated with qualitative platelet defects, e.g. Glanzmann's disease, post-cardiac bypass, uraemia.

Preparation

Platelets may be obtained by harvesting platelet-rich plasma from routinely donated units or by using a cell separator. In general, if the patient is not sensitized to platelet antigens, random donor platelets can be used. The platelet-rich plasma obtained by gentle centrifugation of fresh whole blood is further centrifuged to produce platelet concentrate. If the patient is alloimmunized, an HLA-matched donor is required and the cell separator must be used. Fresh whole blood is a poor source of platelets due to the volumes required.

4.10 Use of blood products

Dosage

From a 500 ml donation of whole blood 1×10^{11} platelets can be harvested. However, 30% of platelets are lost during processing and 30% do not circulate and are sequestered in the spleen.

- Six pooled units of platelet concentrate are given at a time, supplying $3–4 \times 10^{11}$ viable platelets (1×10^{11} is the body's daily production), and this should produce an increment at one hour of $25–35 \times 10^9$/l.
- Platelets should be ABO-compatible although this is not essential.
- Due to red cell contamination rhesus-compatible units should be given to young women.
- In marrow depression platelets should be given daily.
- In bleeding or infection platelet survival is significantly reduced and an increased dosage should be considered.

Storage

Most platelets are given as concentrates, each with a volume of approximately 25 ml, and remain viable up to five days when stored at 22 °C with constant agitation. There is a risk of bacterial contamination. Platelets stored at 4 °C have greater immediate activity but are removed from the circulation very rapidly and have a shorter shelf-life. Platelets can be frozen in 5% DMSO or 12% glycerol and reclaimed as necessary, but the logistics make this unlikely to have wide application.

Complications

Infection. Risks are initially the same as for red cells. However, multiple donors are used, many of the recipients are immunosuppressed, and storage at 22 °C increases the risk of bacterial overgrowth.

Alloimmunization. Platelets contain three antigen systems which may provoke antibody formation:

- HLA.
- Platelet-specific antigens.
- ABO (but not the rhesus system).

Immunization occurs less than would be expected as the recipients are often immunosuppressed, but once it has occurred there is a failure to maintain haemostasis and mild transfusion reactions are seen. Even in the absence of a platelet increment haemostasis may be achieved, but HLA-matched platelets should be given when there is a failure of clinical response.

Granulocyte concentrates

These are used relatively rarely and there are no clear guidelines as to use.

Indications

- Infection in patients with severe neutropenia that has not responded to 24 hours of appropriate antibiotics.
- Shock due to Gram-negative organisms.
- Prophylactic administration is of little or no benefit.

Preparation

Preparation is best achieved using a continuous-flow cell separator, the white cells being separated by differential density centrifugation. Pre-treatment of the donor with corticosteroids increases the circulating pool of granulocytes, and the use of a sedimenting agent such as hydroxyethyl starch aids separation. Granulocytes may be collected by harvesting 'buffy coat' from fresh whole blood but yields are low and benefit is dubious.

Dosage

A daily dose of at least 4×10^{10} cells and preferably 1×10^{11} should be given and continued for at least four days. Intravascular survival is short and there is rarely any granulocyte increment. The cell separator can produce between 5×10^{9} and 5×10^{10} cells in a

2–3 hour procedure. The cells should be given as fresh as possible as they deteriorate rapidly in storage.

Complications

- Infection — in particular cytomegalovirus infections.
- Alloimmunization, usually due to HLA antibodies although specific neutrophil antigens exist (NA, NB).
- Respiratory distress related to aggregates becoming sequestrated in the pulmonary circulation with cough, cyanosis, dyspnoea, fever and rigors. This is particularly a problem when associated with amphotericin infusion.

Donors with chronic granulocytic leukaemia have been used to provide white cells, and although the cells are physiologically and kinetically inferior, the large numbers obtained compensate for this. Patients are rarely available and, as a treatment, leucaphaeresis is inefficient and time-consuming. The use of a donation of malignant cells with the possibility of engraftment and the risk of graft versus host disease from the donated lymphocytes demands that such donations should be irradiated. There is also the risk that the donor, being immunosuppressed, may be harbouring infection.

Plasma products

Platelet-poor plasma can be separated into fresh frozen plasma, cryoprecipitate or stored plasma.

Fresh frozen plasma

Fresh frozen plasma (FFP) is prepared within eight hours of whole blood collection. Each unit is from a single donor, is HBsAg and anti-HIV tested, and contains all the labile coagulation factors. The volume is 200 ml and at −30 °C can be stored for up to 12 months. Where possible ABO-compatible units should be given.

FFP is used for:

- Massive blood transfusion.
- Reversal of oral anticoagulation.

- Hepatic dysfunction.
- Congenital coagulation deficiencies.
- General haemostatic failure, particularly DIC, where all factors may be deficient.
- Occasional replacement fluid in plasma exchange therapy.

Cryoprecipitate

This is produced by freezing freshly separated plasma to −70 °C then thawing at 4 °C. This produces a precipitate which is rich in factors VIII, XIII, fibrinogen and fibronectin. Each unit is prepared from a single donation and contents vary, but each contains 50–100 units of VIII and 0.1–0.3 g of fibrinogen. When refrozen at −30 °C storage life is up to 12 months.

- ABO- and rhesus-compatible units should be used.
- Units should be thawed in a controlled waterbath at 37 °C and given immediately.

Indications include:

- Von Willebrand's disease.
- DIC.
- As fibrinogen replacement in obstetric haemorrhage or following cardiac surgery.

Fibronectin may be valuable in severe trauma and may enhance bacterial phagocytosis but this remains arguable.

Factor VIII and IX concentrates

These concentrates are discussed in the section on haemophilia (p. 265).

Factor VIII is used *only* in the treatment of:

- Haemophilia A.

Factor IX is used principally to treat:

- Haemophilia B.
- Haemophilia A in the presence of inhibitors.
- Reversal of oral anticoagulation.

It can also be used in the management of the rare congenital defects of II, X and for some products, VII.

Factor IX concentrate should *not* be used for:

- Hepatic dysfunction.

or any other haemostatic abnormality without consulting a haematologist. Activated concentrates of factor IX are also available for the treatment of patients with haemophilia A or B who have developed inhibitors. It is uncertain whether these very expensive materials are more effective than unactivated factor IX and their use is reserved for carefully selected cases in large centres.

Salt-poor albumin

This is presented as a 20% solution in bottles containing 20 g. It is reconstituted in 100 ml and is equivalent to 400 ml of PPF. It contains only 20 to 25% of the sodium of PPF. Main uses are:

- Liver disease with severe hypoalbuminaemia and generalized oedema.
- Nephrotic syndrome.

Following infusion, haemodilution occurs rapidly and congestive cardiac failure may be precipitated if renal function is inadequate.

Human albumin solution or plasma protein fraction (PPF)

This is prepared by ethanol fractionation of pooled plasma generally available as a 4% solution and presented in 400 ml volumes. PPF consists of almost 90% albumin. The solution has a physiological sodium content but little potassium or calcium. It is sterilized during preparation and is free of the risk of viral infection. It contains no coagulation factors, blood group antibodies or pseudocholinesterase and can be given irrespective of the blood group. The albumin is used to maintain capillary osmotic pressure and therefore intravascular volume. It may also act as a carrier protein for drugs, enzymes and metabolizers.

Indications:

- Oligaemic shock following haemorrhage.
- Burns.
- Crush injury.

- Plasma exchange replacement fluid.

Combination with a diuretic may mobilize large amounts of tissue fluid when hypoalbuminaemia is the cause of oedema.

Immune globulins

Immune serum globulin is used in the treatment of general immune deficiency states and is used to provide passive prophylaxis against hepatitis A. It contains primarily IgG in the same relative proportions as found in serum. Various monomeric intravenous preparations are becoming available which have similar indications to the i.m. preparations. They appear more effective, probably due to the higher blood levels reached. They also appear to have a novel and unexplained effect in the immune cytopenias (e.g. ITP) in reversing peripheral cellular destruction.

Specific immunoglobulins are available as:

- Anti-rhesus (D) for prophylaxis in rhesus incompatibility to prevent haemolytic disease of the newborn.
- Hepatitis B immune globulin for exposure to contaminated blood in people without evidence of previous hepatitis B infection and the neonates of mothers who are carriers.
- Varicella-zoster IG to prevent or attenuate infection when given within 72 hours of exposure.
- Tetanus IG prepared from individuals immunized to tetanus toxoid.
- IgG preparations against cytomegalovirus, measles, mumps, rubella and rabies.

Some of these preparations should be given to any patient at risk (e.g. rabies) but in general they are particularly appropriate in the immunosuppressed patient.

4.11 Tropical haematology

Malaria

Malaria is caused by four species of the protozoal parasite Plasmodium and is transmitted by female anopheline mosquitos. The disease is widespread in tropical countries including Central and South America, Africa, the Middle East, Asia and the Far East. In the United Kingdom more than 1500 people are diagnosed yearly with approximately 20 deaths. The problem is an increasing one as the malaria-carrying mosquito has become resistant to insecticides and there has developed an increasing resistance to the drugs used to combat the illness. Worldwide deaths number 3.5–5 million a year.

Malaria species

Species	Condition and periodicity
P. vivax	Benign tertian
P. ovale	Ovale tertian
P. malariae	Quartan
P. falciparum	Malignant tertian

Tertian malaria's periodicity is 48 hours, but in falciparum malaria this interval is not always clearly seen. In quartan malaria the symptoms recur every 72 hours.

Life cycle

Within the liver and/or red cells infection and development take place, the parasites appearing in the peripheral blood initially as ring forms. After further development and division (schizogony) merozoites fill the cell, which ruptures, allowing further parasitization of erthrocytes to take place. The cycle is repeated, but eventually gametocytes develop in some red cells. These may be transferred back to the mosquito's stomach following a bite, and fertilization takes place there. Sporogony then occurs and sporozoites are finally released from the salivary glands during feeding to complete the cycle.

In falciparum malaria:

- Schizonts containing merozoites are not usually seen in the peripheral blood as development takes place in the tissues.
- The degree of parasitaemia is variable but important. In the most severe infections up to 20% of red cells may contain parasites.

• There is no secondary exo-erythrocytic stage and this influences treatment.

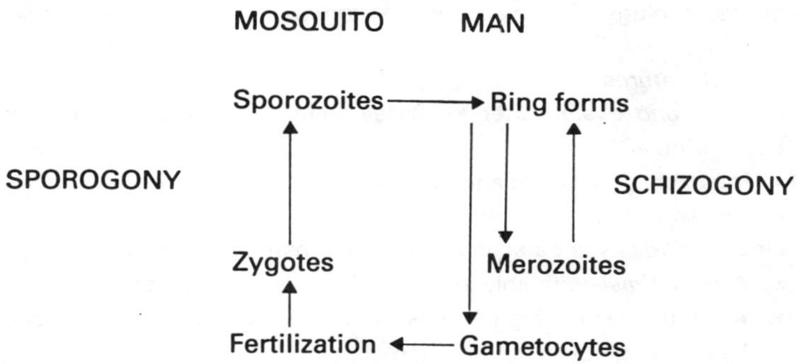

Fig. 4.6 The life cycle in malaria (simplified).

Parasite detection and recognition

Malaria is diagnosed by the detection of parasites in the blood. Thick films are used to identify the presence of parasites because more blood can be examined in 15 minutes' careful study in this way, but experience is necessary for reliable interpretation. Thin films are used to identify the infecting species. The most important distinction is that between *P. falciparum* and the other species, of which the commonest is *P. vivax*. Mixed infections sometimes occur.

Table 4.25 A morphological comparison of *P. vivax* and *P. falciparum*.

	P. vivax	*P. falciparum*
Ring forms	Large irregular	Small and delicate May be more than one ring per cell Rings may have two chromatin dots
	Infestation light	Infestation may be heavy
Schizonts	Contain 12–24 merozoites	Not usually seen in the blood
Gametocytes	Large round	Typical crescent shape

For a full account of the morphology of the various species a larger textbook should be consulted, but Table 4.25 gives a brief guide to the morphology of *P. vivax* and *falciparum*.

Clinical features

P. vivax and ovale. After a 10-day incubation period symptoms begin with:

- Headache, backache and painful limbs.
- Shivering and fever.

Once periodicity is established there are paroxysms in which:

- A *cold phase* with shivering and rigors is followed by
- A *hot phase* with high temperature, nausea, vomiting, headache and a sensation of thirst and then
- A drenching sweat or *wet phase* results in a fall in temperature and return of well-being until the symptoms recur 48 hours later.

This pattern may continue for some weeks, during which mild anaemia develops and the spleen becomes palpable. Eventually the symptoms subside only to return after a few months.

P. malariae malaria has a longer incubation period of a month, periodicity is 72 hours and there are no exo-erythrocytic forms, any recurrence being due to residual infection in the blood.

P. falciparum. The patient falls ill after a 10-day incubation period and remains unwell, the typical periodicity often not becoming established. Symptoms include those described above plus:

- Mental confusion leading to coma and convulsions (cerebral malaria).
- Haemoglobinuria (Blackwater fever).
- Haemoptysis.
- Diarrhoea

and on examination there may be:

- Neurological signs.
- Renal failure.
- Jaundice and pallor.

- A rapidly enlarging liver and spleen.
- Hypotension.

In the laboratory there may be:

- Anaemia.
- Leucopenia.
- Eosinophilia.
- Thrombocytopenia.
- Consumption coagulopathy.

as well as evidence of haemolysis and hepatic and renal dysfunction.

Death may occur from cerebral malaria, renal failure and spontaneous splenic rupture, and is likely to occur in those with the greatest parasitaemia, particularly people travelling into a malarious area without immunity.

- The diagnosis of malaria should be considered in anyone with relevant symptoms who has recently returned from an area where malaria is endemic, especially as immediate treatment may be life-saving in infection with *P. falciparum*.

There are no exo-erythrocytic forms of *P. falciparum* so that relapse does not occur, but failure to eradicate all the blood parasites during treatment may lead to re-emergence of the primary infection.

Mixed infections. Infection by more than one species is not uncommon and may cause daily symptoms or irregular periodicity.

Treatment

Diagnosis and identification of the infecting parasite is important together with an assessment of the severity of the infection, especially in *P. falciparum* infections.

P. vivax and ovale. In adults chloroquine should be given orally:
600 mg initially followed by
300 mg six hours later and then
150 mg twice daily for two days.

If the patient cannot swallow or keep tablets down then a first dose of 200–300 mg may be given i.v. in 250 ml of normal saline followed by a second injection six hours later. i.m. preparations are also available.

Children under 15 years of age are given lower doses, details of which are found in the *British National Formulary* (BNF) and are based on an approximate *total* dose of 30 mg/kg given in divided doses over 4–5 days.

Prevention of relapse is achieved by primaquine 7.5 mg twice daily for 14 days.

- Primaquine should not be given to patients with glucose-6-phosphate dehydrogenase deficiency.

P. malariae. Chloroquine is given as above but primaquine does not need to be added because of the absence of exo-erythrocytic forms.

P. falciparum. Resistance to chloroquine is now widespread in Central and South America, Central and East Afria, India and South-East Asia.

Mildly affected adults may be treated with quinine orally in a dose of 600 mg every eight hours for at least six doses followed by Fansidar (sulphadioxine 500 mg and pyrimethamine 25 mg per tablet) three tablets.

The dosage for children is again given in the BNF.

Seriously ill adults should be treated as shown in Table 4.26. The total dose of quinine should not exceed 2 g over 24 hours. Following the course of quinine Fansidar, three tablets, should be given.

- Infants should not be given quinine intravenously but may be given intramuscular injections in a dose not exceeding 5 mg/kg. As the problem of resistance to chloroquine, quinine and Fansidar increases, alternative drugs are being tried including:
- Quinidine instead of quinine.
- Tetracycline instead of Fansidar.

Table 4.26 Treatment of falciparum malaria.

	Origin of patient	
	Thailand	Elsewhere
Initial quinine dose (as base)	20 mg/kg i.v. over four hours	10 mg/kg i.v. over 2–4 hours
Subsequent doses	10 mg/kg i.v. every eight hours	As above 12-hourly

Advice can be obtained from the centres whose addresses and telephone numbers are given at the end of the section.

Skilled supportive care is important in the management of falciparum malaria.

- Fluid balance must be carefully regulated to avoid overhydration which can lead to pulmonary oedema.
- 5% dextrose may be a preferable infusion fluid for quinine delivery because of the possibility of hypoglycaemia.
- Haemodialysis may be necessary in patients with renal failure.
- Ventilation may be necessary to treat pulmonary oedema or coma.
- Exchange transfusion should be considered, especially if the parasitaemia is greater than 10%.
- Corticosteroids are contraindicated.

Prophylaxis

The prevention of malaria has become increasingly difficult and complex as parasite resistance to drugs has developed. No regimen is guaranteed to prevent malaria, and it is sensible to attempt to avoid mosquito bites, especially after sunset. Precautions include the use of:

- Long-sleeved clothing buttoned at the neck and cuffs with long slacks.

- Mosquito netting, especially if there is no air-conditioning.
- Insect repellants applied liberally to exposed skin.
- Insecticides in the house, particularly at dusk and on retiring.

Stagnant water in the immediate area should be drained if possible. Marshy areas should be avoided.

Tablets should be taken:

- For one week before travelling to a malarious area and
- For six weeks after leaving it.
- *Regularly* as prescribed.

The best drugs to use depend on the area to be visited and current knowledge of resistance patterns. Travellers and their doctors should take advice from the centres listed at the end of the section.

Malarious areas

- *In warm season* (April–October) Egypt, Iran, Iraq, part of Mediterranean.
- *Most of year* India, Pakistan.
- *All year* West, Central and East Africa, Sudan, Central America, Northern half of South America, Panama, Philippines, Indonesia, Burma, Sri Lanka, Malaysia, South-West Pacific.

Leishmaniasis

Visceral leishmaniasis is due to infection with *Leishmania donovani* and is transmitted by sandflies. It is also known as kala-azar. A number of forms have been described, especially:

- Mediterranean — occurring in children and particularly found in the Mediterranean area, China and Latin America. It has an animal reservoir, especially in dogs.
- Indian — without an especially high incidence in children and in which the reservoir of infection is thought to be human.

The main clinical features are:

- Irregular fever and malaise.
- Headache.
- Weight loss.

- Abdominal swelling due to hepatic and splenic enlargement.

In the laboratory:

- Pancytopenia is largely due to hypersplenism but haemolysis and the anaemia of chronic disease contribute to the anaemia.

There is also:

- Hyperglobulinaemia.

The diagnosis is usually made by bone marrow aspiration although splenic puncture may also be performed. Leishman–Donovan bodies are found within macrophages and lying free in the trails. The parasite may also be grown in culture and specific antibodies may be detectable.

- Leishmaniasis occurs in many parts of the world and should be suspected in anyone who has travelled to an endemic area and presents with unexplained splenomegaly, especially if this is associated with fever and pancytopenia.

Management

Sodium stibogluconate is given in a dose of 10 mg/kg daily for 30 days by intramuscular or intravenous injection. The ECG should be regularly monitored as this drug may cause significant dysrhythmias.

Toxoplasmosis

Toxoplasma gondii is protozoal and widely distributed through different species. Two types of disease are produced in man.

Congenital infection

Infected infants suffer from:

- Fever.
- Pallor and jaundice.
- Rash.
- Hepatosplenomegaly.

followed by:

- Neurological disease with retinitis and cerebral calcification.

Adult infection
This is similar to infectious mononucleosis resulting in:
- Fever, rash.
- Lymphadenopathy.
- Hepatosplenomegaly.

but subclinical infection is common.
In the peripheral blood:
- Atypical mononuclear cells

are found and
- Liver function tests are abnormal.

Toxoplasmosis bears marked resemblances to cytomegalovirus infection as well as glandular fever and diagnosis is usually serological, the dye test being most useful. Complement fixation tests may also be used and detect changing antibody patterns.

Management
In the majority of cases no specific treatment is required. The problem of toxoplasmosis in AIDS will not be considered here.

Trypanosomiasis
Three major species of this protozoon are parasitic for man.

African sleeping sickness
Trypanosoma rhodesiense and *T. gambiense* cause sleeping sickness in Africa and are transmitted by tsetse flies. The illness caused by the parasites is very variable in nature and prognosis but the main clinical features are:
- Fever and malaise.
- Lymphadenopathy and splenic enlargement.
- Rash.
- Headache.
- Alteration of consciousness and neurological disturbance.

In the laboratory:
- Parasites may be seen in the peripheral blood, especially in buffy

coat preparations, but the examination of fluid obtained by lymph node puncture may be more rewarding. Fluid should be examined fresh, when parasites may be seen moving between the cells, and in stained films.

There is also:

- Anaemia.
- Monocytosis.
- Hyperglobulinaemia.

Infections due to *T. rhodesiense* are more severe and respond less well to treatment. Control is made difficult by large animal reservoirs of infection.

Chagas' disease

T. cruzi is the cause of American trypanosomiasis or Chagas' disease and is transmitted by reduviid bugs. Most cases occur in South America and Southern Mexico, and as with sleeping sickness there are animal reservoirs.

The infection begins with an erythematous nodule or chagoma followed by:

- Fever.
- Rash.
- Facial oedema.
- Lymphadenopathy and hepatosplenomegaly.

In addition there may be myositis, myocarditis and meningoencephalitis and chronically:

- Megaoesphagus and megacolon due to ganglion nerve cell damage.
- Chronic myocardial disease.

In the laboratory

- Parasites are only occasionally seen in the peripheral blood, the parasite existing mainly in a non-flagellated form in the tissues.

There is also:

- Anaemia.
- Lymphocytosis.

Management of trypanosiamiasis

The treatment of these conditions is difficult and specialist advice should be sought from one of the centres listed below.

Department of Communicable and Tropical Diseases
East Birmingham Hospital
Bordesley Green Road
Birmingham B9 5ST

Tel: 021 772 4311

Liverpool School of Tropical Medicine
Pembroke Place
Liverpool L3 5QA

Tel: 051 708 9393

Hospital for Tropical Diseases
4 St. Pancras Way
London NW1 OPE

Tel: 01 387 4411

Ross Institute of Tropical Hygiene
London Shcool of Hygiene and Tropical Medicine
Keppel Street
London WC1E 7HT

Tel: 01 636 8636

Travellers may also contact:

Department of Health and Social Security
Alexander Fleming House
Elephant and Castle
London SE1 6BY

Tel: 01 407 5522

Useful addresses

Anthony Nolan Bone Marrow Appeal
St. Mary Abbots Hospital
Marloes Road, Kensington
London W8 5LQ

Tel: 01 937 2660

BACUP (British Association of Cancer United Patients)
121/123 Charterhouse Street
London EC1M 64A

Tel: 01 608 1661

Cancer Aftercare and Rehabilitation Society
Lodge Cottage
Church Lane
Timsbury
Bath

Tel: 0761 70731

Cancer Relief
Michael Sobell House
30 Dorset Square
London NW1 6QL

Tel: 01 402 8125

Cypriot (Greek) Advisory Service
26 Crowndale Road
London NW1 1TT

Tel: 01 388 7971/2

Cyprus Turkish Association
34/35 D'Arblay Street
London W1A 4YL

Tel: 01 437 4940

Useful addresses

The Haemophilia Society
125 Westminster Bridge Road
London SE1 7HR

Tel: 01 928 2020

Leukaemia Research Fund
43 Great Ormond Street
London WC1N 3JJ

Tel: 01 405 0101

Leukaemia Society
P.O. Box 82
Exeter EX2 5DP

Tel: 0392 218514

Marie Curie Memorial Foundation
28 Belgrave Square
London SW1X 8QG

Tel: 01 235 3325

Organisation of Sickle Cell Anaemia (OSCAR)
200A High Road
Wood Green
London N22

Tel: 01 889 3300 or 01 889 4844

The Sickle Cell Society
c/o Brent Community Health Council
16 High Street
Harlesden
London NW10 4LX

Tel: 01 451 3293

Useful addresses

Terrence Higgins Trust
BM AIDS
London WC1N 3XX

Tel: 01 833 2971 (help-line open 7–10 p.m. Mon-Fri, 3–10 p.m. Sat-Sun)

United Kingdom Thalassaemia Society
107 Nightingale Lane
London N8

Tel: 01 384 0437

Normal ranges and average normal values

Basic haematology

Value	Infant	Child	Adult	
			Male	Female
Haemoglobin concentration (g/dl)	14.0–22.0	12.0	13.0–18.0	12.0–16.0
Red cells $\times 10^{12}$/l	4.0– 6.0	4.5	4.5– 6.5	3.9– 5.6
Haematocrit (PVC)	0.5– 0.7	0.4	0.4–0.54	0.37–0.47
MCV (fl)	106	80	76–96	
MCH (pg)			27–32	
MCHC (g/dl)			32–36	
Reticulocytes (%)			<2	
White cells $\times 10^{9}$/l	10.0–25.0	5.0–15.0	4.0–11.0	
Neutrophils		2.0– 6.0	2.0– 7.5	
Lymphocytes		5.5– 8.5	1.5– 4.0	
Monocytes		0.7– 1.5	0.2– 0.8	
Eosinophils		0.3– 0.8	Up to 0.4	
Basophils		<0.1	<0.1	
Platelets $\times 10^{9}$/l			150–400	
ESR (mm in one hour)			0–5	0–7

Haemoglobins

Type	Neonate	Adult
Haemoglobin A (%)	30	97
F (%)	70	<1
A_2(%)	<1	1.5–3.0

Haematinics

	Adults
Plasma iron (µmol/l)	13–32
Total iron binding capacity (TIBC) (µmol/l)	47–70
Ferritin (µg/l)	25–400
Vitamin B_{12} (ng/l)	210–920
Serum folate (µg/l)	2–14
Red cell folate (µg/l)	125–600

Haemostasis

Platelet count $\times 10^9$/l	150–400
Bleeding time (template)	Up to 9 minutes
Prothrombin ratio	1.0–1.3
Partial thromboplastin time (KCCT) (secs)	36–48
Thrombin time (secs)	10–12
Fibrinogen concentration (g/l)	2–4
Euglobulin lysis time (hours)	>2
Fibrinogen degradation products (mg/l)	<10
Antithrombin III (i.u./dl)	80–120

Miscellaneous

Haptoglobins (g/l)	0.9–3.8
Red cell mass (ml/kg)	
Male	26–33
Female	22–29
Neutrophil alkaline phosphatase per 100 neutrophils	30–180

Index

Index

Index

Index

Index

Index

Index

Index

Index

Index

Index

Index